50% OFF
Online CSCS® Prep Course!

Dear Customer,

Thank you for your purchase of this CSCS Study Guide. Included with your purchase is **discounted access to our online CSCS Prep Course**. Many CSCS courses are needlessly expensive and don't deliver enough value. Our course provides the best CSCS prep material, and with discounted access, **you only pay half price**.

We have structured our online course to perfectly complement your printed study guide. The CSCS Prep Course contains **in-depth lessons** that cover all the most important topics, over **1,300 practice questions** to ensure you feel prepared, and more than **250 digital flashcards**, so you can study while you're on the go.

Online CSCS Prep Course

Topics Included:

- Exercise Sciences
- Sport Psychology
- Nutrition
- Exercise Technique
- Program Design
- Organization and Administration
- Program Implementation

Course Features:

- CSCS Study Guide
  - Get content that complements our best-selling study guide.
- Full-Length Practice Tests
  - With over 1,300 practice questions, you can test yourself again and again.
- Mobile Friendly
  - If you need to study on the go, the course is easily accessible from your mobile device.
- CSCS Flashcards
  - Our course includes a flashcard mode with over 250 content cards to help you study.

To lock in your discounted access, visit mometrix.com/university/cscs or simply scan this QR code with your smartphone. At the checkout page, enter the discount code: **cscs50off**

If you have any questions or concerns, please contact us at support@mometrix.com.

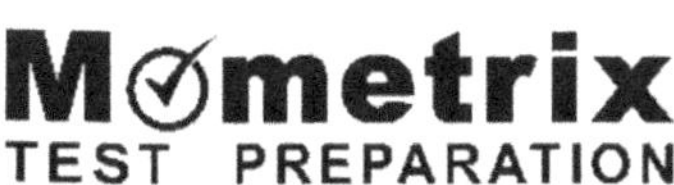

Access Your Online Resources

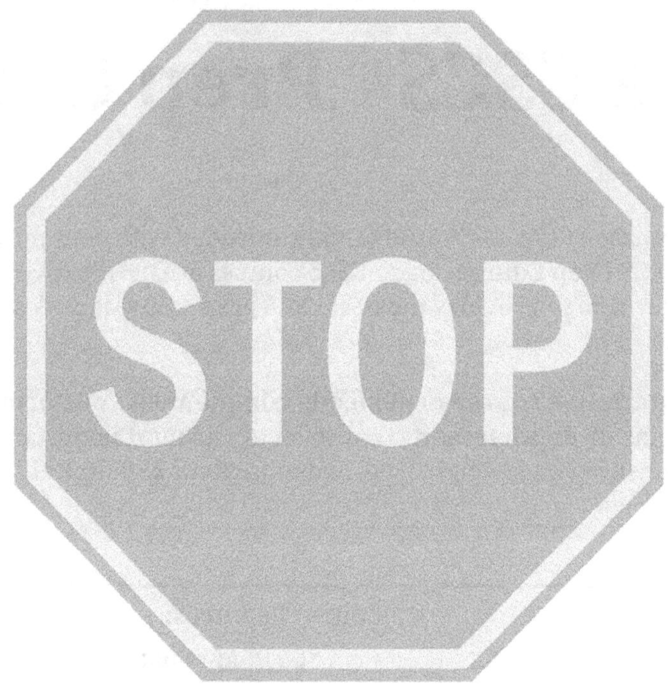

Don't miss out on the Online Resources included with your purchase!

Your purchase of this product unlocks access to our Online Resources page. Elevate your study experience with our **interactive practice test interface**, along with all of the additional resources that we couldn't include in this book.

Flip to the Online Resources section at the end of this book to find the link and a QR code to get started!

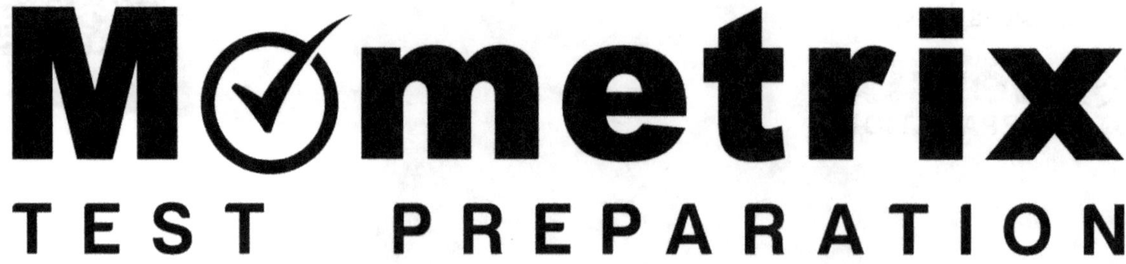

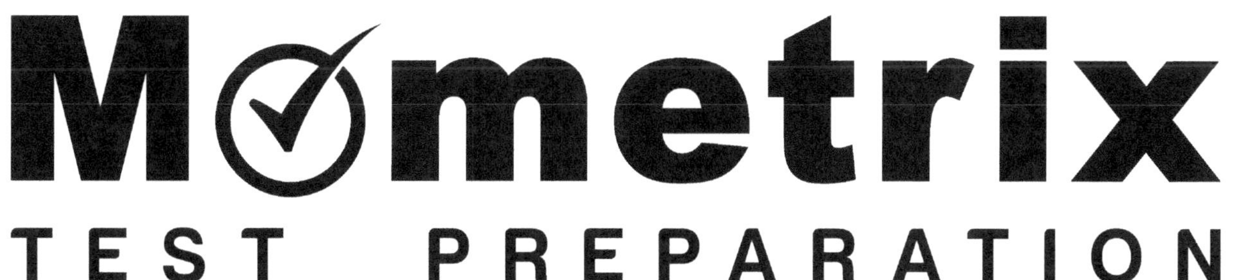

CSCS®

Study Guide 2026-2027

2 Full-Length Practice Tests

Secrets Exam Prep Book for the NSCA® Certified Strength and Conditioning Specialist Assessment

4th Edition

Written and edited by Matthew Bowling

Printed in the United States of America

This paper meets the requirements of ANSI/NISO Z39.48-1992 (Permanence of Paper).

Paperback
ISBN 13: 978-1-5167-3157-2
ISBN 10: 1-5167-3157-3

DEAR FUTURE EXAM SUCCESS STORY

First of all, **THANK YOU** for purchasing Mometrix study materials!

Second, congratulations! You are one of the few determined test-takers who are committed to doing whatever it takes to excel on your exam. **You have come to the right place.** We developed these study materials with one goal in mind: to deliver you the information you need in a format that's concise and easy to use.

In addition to optimizing your guide for the content of the test, we've outlined our recommended steps for breaking down the preparation process into small, attainable goals so you can make sure you stay on track.

We've also analyzed the entire test-taking process, identifying the most common pitfalls and showing how you can overcome them and be ready for any curveball the test throws you.

Standardized testing is one of the biggest obstacles on your road to success, which only increases the importance of doing well in the high-pressure, high-stakes environment of test day. Your results on this test could have a significant impact on your future, and this guide provides the information and practical advice to help you achieve your full potential on test day.

Your success is our success

We would love to hear from you! If you would like to share the story of your exam success or if you have any questions or comments in regard to our products, please contact us at **800-673-8175** or **support@mometrix.com**.

Thanks again for your business and we wish you continued success!

Sincerely,
The Mometrix Test Preparation Team

Need more help? Check out our flashcards at:
http://mometrixflashcards.com/CSCS

Written and edited by the Mometrix Exam Secrets Test Prep Team
Printed in the United States of America

TABLE OF CONTENTS

Introduction

Thank you for purchasing this resource! You have made the choice to prepare yourself for a test that could have a huge impact on your future, and this guide is designed to help you be fully ready for test day. Obviously, it's important to have a solid understanding of the test material, but you also need to be prepared for the unique environment and stressors of the test, so that you can perform to the best of your abilities.

For this purpose, the first section that appears in this guide is the **Secret Keys**. We've devoted countless hours to meticulously researching what works and what doesn't, and we've boiled down our findings to the five most impactful steps you can take to improve your performance on the test. We start at the beginning with study planning and move through the preparation process, all the way to the testing strategies that will help you get the most out of what you know when you're finally sitting in front of the test.

We recommend that you start preparing for your test as far in advance as possible. However, if you've bought this guide as a last-minute study resource and only have a few days before your test, we recommend that you skip over the first two Secret Keys since they address a long-term study plan.

If you struggle with **test anxiety**, we strongly encourage you to check out our recommendations for how you can overcome it. Test anxiety is a formidable foe, but it can be beaten, and we want to make sure you have the tools you need to defeat it.

Secret Key #1 – Plan Big, Study Small

There's a lot riding on your performance. If you want to ace this test, you're going to need to keep your skills sharp and the material fresh in your mind. You need a plan that lets you review everything you need to know while still fitting in your schedule. We'll break this strategy down into three categories.

Information Organization

Start with the information you already have: the official test outline. From this, you can make a complete list of all the concepts you need to cover before the test. Organize these concepts into groups that can be studied together, and create a list of any related vocabulary you need to learn so you can brush up on any difficult terms. You'll want to keep this vocabulary list handy once you actually start studying since you may need to add to it along the way.

Time Management

Once you have your set of study concepts, decide how to spread them out over the time you have left before the test. Break your study plan into small, clear goals so you have a manageable task for each day and know exactly what you're doing. Then just focus on one small step at a time. When you manage your time this way, you don't need to spend hours at a time studying. Studying a small block of content for a short period each day helps you retain information better and avoid stressing over how much you have left to do. You can relax knowing that you have a plan to cover everything in time. In order for this strategy to be effective though, you have to start studying early and stick to your schedule. Avoid the exhaustion and futility that comes from last-minute cramming!

Study Environment

The environment you study in has a big impact on your learning. Studying in a coffee shop, while probably more enjoyable, is not likely to be as fruitful as studying in a quiet room. It's important to keep distractions to a minimum. You're only planning to study for a short block of time, so make the most of it. Don't pause to check your phone or get up to find a snack. It's also important to **avoid multitasking**. Research has consistently shown that multitasking will make your studying dramatically less effective. Your study area should also be comfortable and well-lit so you don't have the distraction of straining your eyes or sitting on an uncomfortable chair.

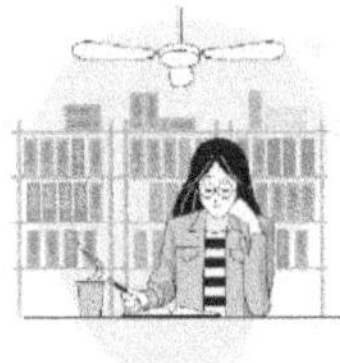

The time of day you study is also important. You want to be rested and alert. Don't wait until just before bedtime. Study when you'll be most likely to comprehend and remember. Even better, if you know what time of day your test will be, set that time aside for study. That way your brain will be used to working on that subject at that specific time and you'll have a better chance of recalling information.

Finally, it can be helpful to team up with others who are studying for the same test. Your actual studying should be done in as isolated an environment as possible, but the work of organizing the information and setting up the study plan can be divided up. In between study sessions, you can discuss with your teammates the concepts that you're all studying and quiz each other on the details. Just be sure that your teammates are as serious about the test as you are. If you find that your study time is being replaced with social time, you might need to find a new team.

Secret Key #2 – Make Your Studying Count

You're devoting a lot of time and effort to preparing for this test, so you want to be absolutely certain it will pay off. This means doing more than just reading the content and hoping you can remember it on test day. It's important to make every minute of study count. There are two main areas you can focus on to make your studying count.

Retention

It doesn't matter how much time you study if you can't remember the material. You need to make sure you are retaining the concepts. To check your retention of the information you're learning, try recalling it at later times with minimal prompting. Try carrying around flashcards and glance at one or two from time to time or ask a friend who's also studying for the test to quiz you.

To enhance your retention, look for ways to put the information into practice so that you can apply it rather than simply recalling it. If you're using the information in practical ways, it will be much easier to remember. Similarly, it helps to solidify a concept in your mind if you're not only reading it to yourself but also explaining it to someone else. Ask a friend to let you teach them about a concept you're a little shaky on (or speak aloud to an imaginary audience if necessary). As you try to summarize, define, give examples, and answer your friend's questions, you'll understand the concepts better and they will stay with you longer. Finally, step back for a big picture view and ask yourself how each piece of information fits with the whole subject. When you link the different concepts together and see them working together as a whole, it's easier to remember the individual components.

Finally, practice showing your work on any multi-step problems, even if you're just studying. Writing out each step you take to solve a problem will help solidify the process in your mind, and you'll be more likely to remember it during the test.

Modality

Modality simply refers to the means or method by which you study. Choosing a study modality that fits your own individual learning style is crucial. No two people learn best in exactly the same way, so it's important to know your strengths and use them to your advantage.

For example, if you learn best by visualization, focus on visualizing a concept in your mind and draw an image or a diagram. Try color-coding your notes, illustrating them, or creating symbols that will trigger your mind to recall a learned concept. If you learn best by hearing or discussing information, find a study partner who learns the same way or read aloud to yourself. Think about how to put the information in your own words. Imagine that you are giving a lecture on the topic and record yourself so you can listen to it later.

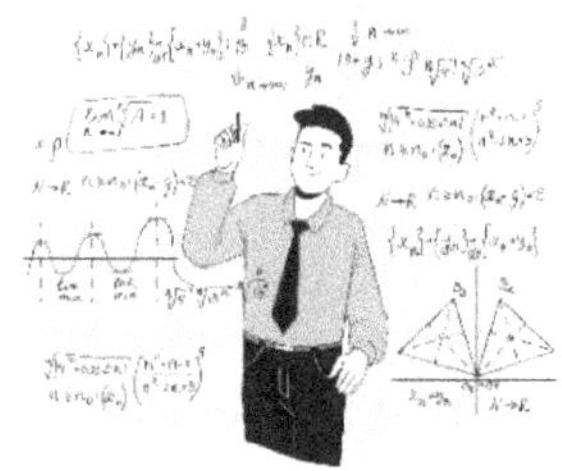

For any learning style, flashcards can be helpful. Organize the information so you can take advantage of spare moments to review. Underline key words or phrases. Use different colors for different categories. Mnemonic devices (such as creating a short list in which every item starts with the same letter) can also help with retention. Find what works best for you and use it to store the information in your mind most effectively and easily.

Secret Key #3 – Practice the Right Way

Your success on test day depends not only on how many hours you put into preparing, but also on whether you prepared the right way. It's good to check along the way to see if your studying is paying off. One of the most effective ways to do this is by taking practice tests to evaluate your progress. Practice tests are useful because they show exactly where you need to improve. Every time you take a practice test, pay special attention to these three groups of questions:

- The questions you got wrong
- The questions you had to guess on, even if you guessed right
- The questions you found difficult or slow to work through

This will show you exactly what your weak areas are, and where you need to devote more study time. Ask yourself why each of these questions gave you trouble. Was it because you didn't understand the material? Was it because you didn't remember the vocabulary? Do you need more repetitions on this type of question to build speed and confidence? Dig into those questions and figure out how you can strengthen your weak areas as you go back to review the material.

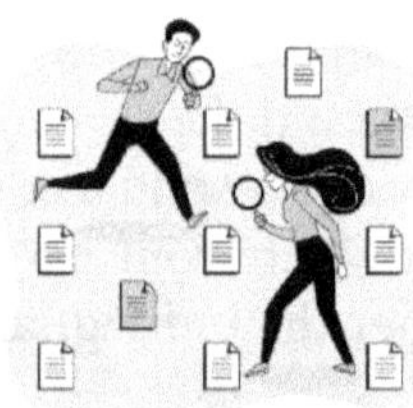

Additionally, many practice tests have a section explaining the answer choices. It can be tempting to read the explanation and think that you now have a good understanding of the concept. However, an explanation likely only covers part of the question's broader context. Even if the explanation makes perfect sense, **go back and investigate** every concept related to the question until you're positive you have a thorough understanding.

As you go along, keep in mind that the practice test is just that: practice. Memorizing these questions and answers will not be very helpful on the actual test because it is unlikely to have any of the same exact questions. If you only know the right answers to the sample questions, you won't be prepared for the real thing. **Study the concepts** until you understand them fully, and then you'll be able to answer any question that shows up on the test.

It's important to wait on the practice tests until you're ready. If you take a test on your first day of study, you may be overwhelmed by the amount of material covered and how much you need to learn. Work up to it gradually.

On test day, you'll need to be prepared for answering questions, managing your time, and using the test-taking strategies you've learned. It's a lot to balance, like a mental marathon that will have a big impact on your future. Like training for a marathon, you'll need to start slowly and work your way up. When test day arrives, you'll be ready.

Start with the strategies you've read in the first two Secret Keys—plan your course and study in the way that works best for you. If you have time, consider using multiple study resources to get different approaches to the same concepts. It can be helpful to see difficult concepts from more than one angle. Then find a good source for practice tests. Many times, the test website will suggest potential study resources or provide sample tests.

Practice Test Strategy

If you're able to find at least three practice tests, we recommend this strategy:

Untimed and Open-Book Practice

Take the first test with no time constraints and with your notes and study guide handy. Take your time and focus on applying the strategies you've learned.

Timed and Open-Book Practice

Take the second practice test open-book as well, but set a timer and practice pacing yourself to finish in time.

Timed and Closed-Book Practice

Take any other practice tests as if it were test day. Set a timer and put away your study materials. Sit at a table or desk in a quiet room, imagine yourself at the testing center, and answer questions as quickly and accurately as possible.

Keep repeating timed and closed-book tests on a regular basis until you run out of practice tests or it's time for the actual test. Your mind will be ready for the schedule and stress of test day, and you'll be able to focus on recalling the material you've learned.

Secret Key #4 – Pace Yourself

Once you're fully prepared for the material on the test, your biggest challenge on test day will be managing your time. Just knowing that the clock is ticking can make you panic even if you have plenty of time left. Work on pacing yourself so you can build confidence against the time constraints of the exam. Pacing is a difficult skill to master, especially in a high-pressure environment, so **practice is vital.**

Set time expectations for your pace based on how much time is available. For example, if a section has 60 questions and the time limit is 30 minutes, you know you have to average 30 seconds or less per question in order to answer them all. Although 30 seconds is the hard limit, set 25 seconds per question as your goal, so you reserve extra time to spend on harder questions. When you budget extra time for the harder questions, you no longer have any reason to stress when those questions take longer to answer.

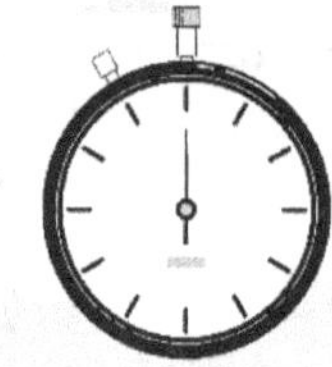

Don't let this time expectation distract you from working through the test at a calm, steady pace, but keep it in mind so you don't spend too much time on any one question. Recognize that taking extra time on one question you don't understand may keep you from answering two that you do understand later in the test. If your time limit for a question is up and you're still not sure of the answer, mark it and move on, and come back to it later if the time and the test format allow. If the testing format doesn't allow you to return to earlier questions, just make an educated guess; then put it out of your mind and move on.

On the easier questions, be careful not to rush. It may seem wise to hurry through them so you have more time for the challenging ones, but it's not worth missing one if you know the concept and just didn't take the time to read the question fully. Work efficiently but make sure you understand the question and have looked at all of the answer choices, since more than one may seem right at first.

Even if you're paying attention to the time, you may find yourself a little behind at some point. You should speed up to get back on track, but do so wisely. Don't panic; just take a few seconds less on each question until you're caught up. Don't guess without thinking, but do look through the answer choices and eliminate any you know are wrong. If you can get down to two choices, it is often worthwhile to guess from those. Once you've chosen an answer, move on and don't dwell on any that you skipped or had to hurry through. If a question was taking too long, chances are it was one of the harder ones, so you weren't as likely to get it right anyway.

On the other hand, if you find yourself getting ahead of schedule, it may be beneficial to slow down a little. The more quickly you work, the more likely you are to make a careless mistake that will affect your score. You've budgeted time for each question, so don't be afraid to spend that time. Practice an efficient but careful pace to get the most out of the time you have.

Secret Key #5 – Have a Plan for Guessing

When you're taking the test, you may find yourself stuck on a question. Some of the answer choices seem better than others, but you don't see the one answer choice that is obviously correct. What do you do?

The scenario described above is very common, yet most test takers have not effectively prepared for it. Developing and practicing a plan for guessing may be one of the single most effective uses of your time as you get ready for the exam.

In developing your plan for guessing, there are three questions to address:

- When should you start the guessing process?
- How should you narrow down the choices?
- Which answer should you choose?

When to Start the Guessing Process

Unless your plan for guessing is to select C every time (which, despite its merits, is not what we recommend), you need to leave yourself enough time to apply your answer elimination strategies. Since you have a limited amount of time for each question, that means that if you're going to give yourself the best shot at guessing correctly, you have to decide quickly whether or not you will guess.

Of course, the best-case scenario is that you don't have to guess at all, so first, see if you can answer the question based on your knowledge of the subject and basic reasoning skills. Focus on the key words in the question and try to jog your memory of related topics. Give yourself a chance to bring the knowledge to mind, but once you realize that you don't have (or you can't access) the knowledge you need to answer the question, it's time to start the guessing process.

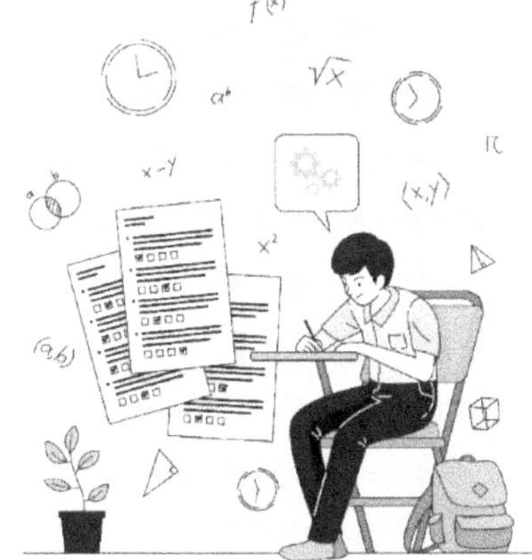

It's almost always better to start the guessing process too early than too late. It only takes a few seconds to remember something and answer the question from knowledge. Carefully eliminating wrong answer choices takes longer. Plus, going through the process of eliminating answer choices can actually help jog your memory.

Summary: Start the guessing process as soon as you decide that you can't answer the question based on your knowledge.

How to Narrow Down the Choices

The next chapter in this book (**Test-Taking Strategies**) includes a wide range of strategies for how to approach questions and how to look for answer choices to eliminate. You will definitely want to read those carefully, practice them, and figure out which ones work best for you. Here though, we're going to address a mindset rather than a particular strategy.

Your odds of guessing an answer correctly depend on how many options you are choosing from.

Number of options left	5	4	3	2	1
Odds of guessing correctly	20%	25%	33%	50%	100%

You can see from this chart just how valuable it is to be able to eliminate incorrect answers and make an educated guess, but there are two things that many test takers do that cause them to miss out on the benefits of guessing:

- Accidentally eliminating the correct answer
- Selecting an answer based on an impression

We'll look at the first one here, and the second one in the next section.

To avoid accidentally eliminating the correct answer, we recommend a thought exercise called **the $5 challenge**. In this challenge, you only eliminate an answer choice from contention if you are willing to bet $5 on it being wrong. Why $5? Five dollars is a small but not insignificant amount of money. It's an amount you could afford to lose but wouldn't want to throw away. And while losing $5 once might not hurt too much, doing it twenty times will set you back $100. In the same way, each small decision you make—eliminating a choice here, guessing on a question there—won't by itself impact your score very much, but when you put them all together, they can make a big difference. By holding each answer choice elimination decision to a higher standard, you can reduce the risk of accidentally eliminating the correct answer.

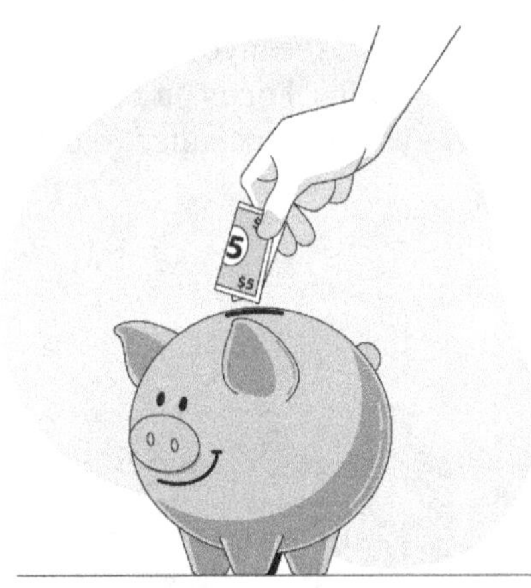

The $5 challenge can also be applied in a positive sense: If you are willing to bet $5 that an answer choice *is* correct, go ahead and mark it as correct.

Summary: Only eliminate an answer choice if you are willing to bet $5 that it is wrong.

Which Answer to Choose

You're taking the test. You've run into a hard question and decided you'll have to guess. You've eliminated all the answer choices you're willing to bet $5 on. Now you have to pick an answer. Why do we even need to talk about this? Why can't you just pick whichever one you feel like when the time comes?

The answer to these questions is that if you don't come into the test with a plan, you'll rely on your impression to select an answer choice, and if you do that, you risk falling into a trap. The test writers know that everyone who takes their test will be guessing on some of the questions, so they intentionally write wrong answer choices to seem plausible. You still have to pick an answer though, and if the wrong answer choices are designed to look right, how can you ever be sure that you're not falling for their trap? The best solution we've found to this dilemma is to take the decision out of your hands entirely. Here is the process we recommend:

Once you've eliminated any choices that you are confident (willing to bet $5) are wrong, select the first remaining choice as your answer.

Whether you choose to select the first remaining choice, the second, or the last, the important thing is that you use some preselected standard. Using this approach guarantees that you will not be enticed into selecting an answer choice that looks right, because you are not basing your decision on how the answer choices look.

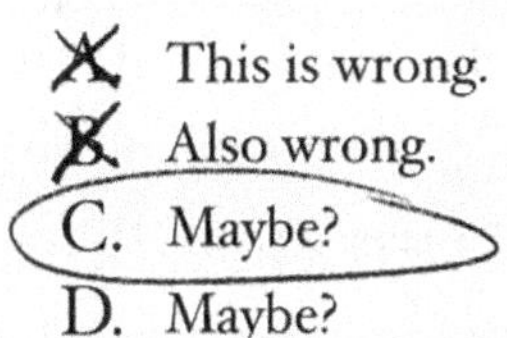

This is not meant to make you question your knowledge. Instead, it is to help you recognize the difference between your knowledge and your impressions. There's a huge difference between thinking an answer is right because of what you know, and thinking an answer is right because it looks or sounds like it should be right.

Summary: To ensure that your selection is appropriately random, make a predetermined selection from among all answer choices you have not eliminated.

Test-Taking Strategies

This section contains a list of test-taking strategies that you may find helpful as you work through the test. By taking what you know and applying logical thought, you can maximize your chances of answering any question correctly!

It is very important to realize that every question is different and every person is different: no single strategy will work on every question, and no single strategy will work for every person. That's why we've included all of them here, so you can try them out and determine which ones work best for different types of questions and which ones work best for you.

Question Strategies

✓ Read Carefully

Read the question and the answer choices carefully. Don't miss the question because you misread the terms. You have plenty of time to read each question thoroughly and make sure you understand what is being asked. Yet a happy medium must be attained, so don't waste too much time. You must read carefully and efficiently.

✓ Contextual Clues

Look for contextual clues. If the question includes a word you are not familiar with, look at the immediate context for some indication of what the word might mean. Contextual clues can often give you all the information you need to decipher the meaning of an unfamiliar word. Even if you can't determine the meaning, you may be able to narrow down the possibilities enough to make a solid guess at the answer to the question.

✓ Prefixes

If you're having trouble with a word in the question or answer choices, try dissecting it. Take advantage of every clue that the word might include. Prefixes can be a huge help. Usually, they allow you to determine a basic meaning. *Pre-* means before, *post-* means after, *pro-* is positive, *de-* is negative. From prefixes, you can get an idea of the general meaning of the word and try to put it into context.

✓ Hedge Words

Watch out for critical hedge words, such as *likely, may, can, often, almost, mostly, usually, generally, rarely*, and *sometimes*. Question writers insert these hedge phrases to cover every possibility. Often an answer choice will be wrong simply because it leaves no room for exception. Be on guard for answer choices that have definitive words such as *exactly* and *always*.

✓ Switchback Words

Stay alert for *switchbacks*. These are the words and phrases frequently used to alert you to shifts in thought. The most common switchback words are *but, although*, and *however*. Others include *nevertheless, on the other hand, even though, while, in spite of, despite*, and *regardless of*. Switchback words are important to catch because they can change the direction of the question or an answer choice.

⊘ Face Value

When in doubt, use common sense. Accept the situation in the problem at face value. Don't read too much into it. These problems will not require you to make wild assumptions. If you have to go beyond creativity and warp time or space in order to have an answer choice fit the question, then you should move on and consider the other answer choices. These are normal problems rooted in reality. The applicable relationship or explanation may not be readily apparent, but it is there for you to figure out. Use your common sense to interpret anything that isn't clear.

Answer Choice Strategies

⊘ Answer Selection

The most thorough way to pick an answer choice is to identify and eliminate wrong answers until only one is left, then confirm it is the correct answer. Sometimes an answer choice may immediately seem right, but be careful. The test writers will usually put more than one reasonable answer choice on each question, so take a second to read all of them and make sure that the other choices are not equally obvious. As long as you have time left, it is better to read every answer choice than to pick the first one that looks right without checking the others.

⊘ Answer Choice Families

An answer choice family consists of two (in rare cases, three) answer choices that are very similar in construction and cannot all be true at the same time. If you see two answer choices that are direct opposites or parallels, one of them is usually the correct answer. For instance, if one answer choice says that quantity x increases and another either says that quantity x decreases (opposite) or says that quantity y increases (parallel), then those answer choices would fall into the same family. An answer choice that doesn't match the construction of the answer choice family is more likely to be incorrect. Most questions will not have answer choice families, but when they do appear, you should be prepared to recognize them.

⊘ Eliminate Answers

Eliminate answer choices as soon as you realize they are wrong, but make sure you consider all possibilities. If you are eliminating answer choices and realize that the last one you are left with is also wrong, don't panic. Start over and consider each choice again. There may be something you missed the first time that you will realize on the second pass.

⊘ Avoid Fact Traps

Don't be distracted by an answer choice that is factually true but doesn't answer the question. You are looking for the choice that answers the question. Stay focused on what the question is asking for so you don't accidentally pick an answer that is true but incorrect. Always go back to the question and make sure the answer choice you've selected actually answers the question and is not merely a true statement.

⊘ Extreme Statements

In general, you should avoid answers that put forth extreme actions as standard practice or proclaim controversial ideas as established fact. An answer choice that states the "process should be used in certain situations, if..." is much more likely to be correct than one that states the "process should be discontinued completely." The first is a calm rational statement and doesn't even make a definitive, uncompromising stance, using a hedge word *if* to provide wiggle room, whereas the second choice is far more extreme.

⊘ BENCHMARK

As you read through the answer choices and you come across one that seems to answer the question well, mentally select that answer choice. This is not your final answer, but it's the one that will help you evaluate the other answer choices. The one that you selected is your benchmark or standard for judging each of the other answer choices. Every other answer choice must be compared to your benchmark. That choice is correct until proven otherwise by another answer choice beating it. If you find a better answer, then that one becomes your new benchmark. Once you've decided that no other choice answers the question as well as your benchmark, you have your final answer.

⊘ PREDICT THE ANSWER

Before you even start looking at the answer choices, it is often best to try to predict the answer. When you come up with the answer on your own, it is easier to avoid distractions and traps because you will know exactly what to look for. The right answer choice is unlikely to be word-for-word what you came up with, but it should be a close match. Even if you are confident that you have the right answer, you should still take the time to read each option before moving on.

General Strategies

⊘ TOUGH QUESTIONS

If you are stumped on a problem or it appears too hard or too difficult, don't waste time. Move on! Remember though, if you can quickly check for obviously incorrect answer choices, your chances of guessing correctly are greatly improved. Before you completely give up, at least try to knock out a couple of possible answers. Eliminate what you can and then guess at the remaining answer choices before moving on.

⊘ CHECK YOUR WORK

Since you will probably not know every term listed and the answer to every question, it is important that you get credit for the ones that you do know. Don't miss any questions through careless mistakes. If at all possible, try to take a second to look back over your answer selection and make sure you've selected the correct answer choice and haven't made a costly careless mistake (such as marking an answer choice that you didn't mean to mark). This quick double check should more than pay for itself in caught mistakes for the time it costs.

⊘ PACE YOURSELF

It's easy to be overwhelmed when you're looking at a page full of questions; your mind is confused and full of random thoughts, and the clock is ticking down faster than you would like. Calm down and maintain the pace that you have set for yourself. Especially as you get down to the last few minutes of the test, don't let the small numbers on the clock make you panic. As long as you are on track by monitoring your pace, you are guaranteed to have time for each question.

⊘ DON'T RUSH

It is very easy to make errors when you are in a hurry. Maintaining a fast pace in answering questions is pointless if it makes you miss questions that you would have gotten right otherwise. Test writers like to include distracting information and wrong answers that seem right. Taking a little extra time to avoid careless mistakes can make all the difference in your test score. Find a pace that allows you to be confident in the answers that you select.

✅ KEEP MOVING

Panicking will not help you pass the test, so do your best to stay calm and keep moving. Taking deep breaths and going through the answer elimination steps you practiced can help to break through a stress barrier and keep your pace.

Final Notes

The combination of a solid foundation of content knowledge and the confidence that comes from practicing your plan for applying that knowledge is the key to maximizing your performance on test day. As your foundation of content knowledge is built up and strengthened, you'll find that the strategies included in this chapter become more and more effective in helping you quickly sift through the distractions and traps of the test to isolate the correct answer.

Now that you're preparing to move forward into the test content chapters of this book, be sure to keep your goal in mind. As you read, think about how you will be able to apply this information on the test. If you've already seen sample questions for the test and you have an idea of the question format and style, try to come up with questions of your own that you can answer based on what you're reading. This will give you valuable practice applying your knowledge in the same ways you can expect to on test day.

Good luck and good studying!

Exercise Sciences

Muscle Anatomy and Physiology

Skeletal Muscle Anatomy

Skeletal muscle is made up of long, cylindrical muscle fibers, also known as muscle cells. These fibers are grouped into bundles known as **fasciculi.** There are three types of connective tissue that subdivide skeletal muscle.

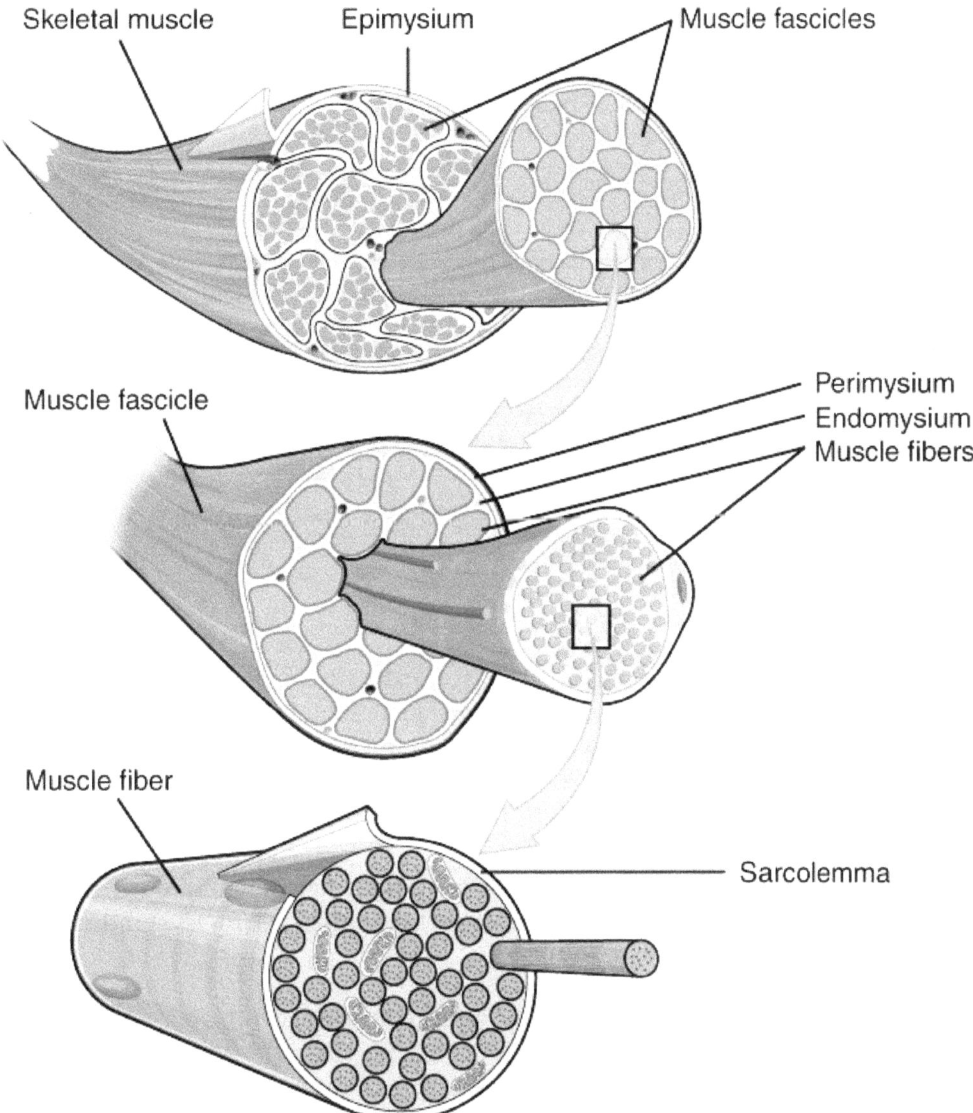

The largest layer is the **epimysium**, which surrounds the entire muscle in a sheath of fibrous connective tissue. The next layer is the **perimysium**, which covers the fascicles, or grouped bundles of muscle fibers. The **sarcolemma** is the cell membrane further surrounding each muscle fiber, and the **endomysium** underneath the sarcolemma surrounds each individual muscle fiber within the muscle. The interior of each individual muscle fiber, the **sarcoplasm,** contains small structures called **myofibrils.** Each myofibril is made up of even smaller structures called **myofilaments**, which are the contractile components whose action initiates muscle movement.

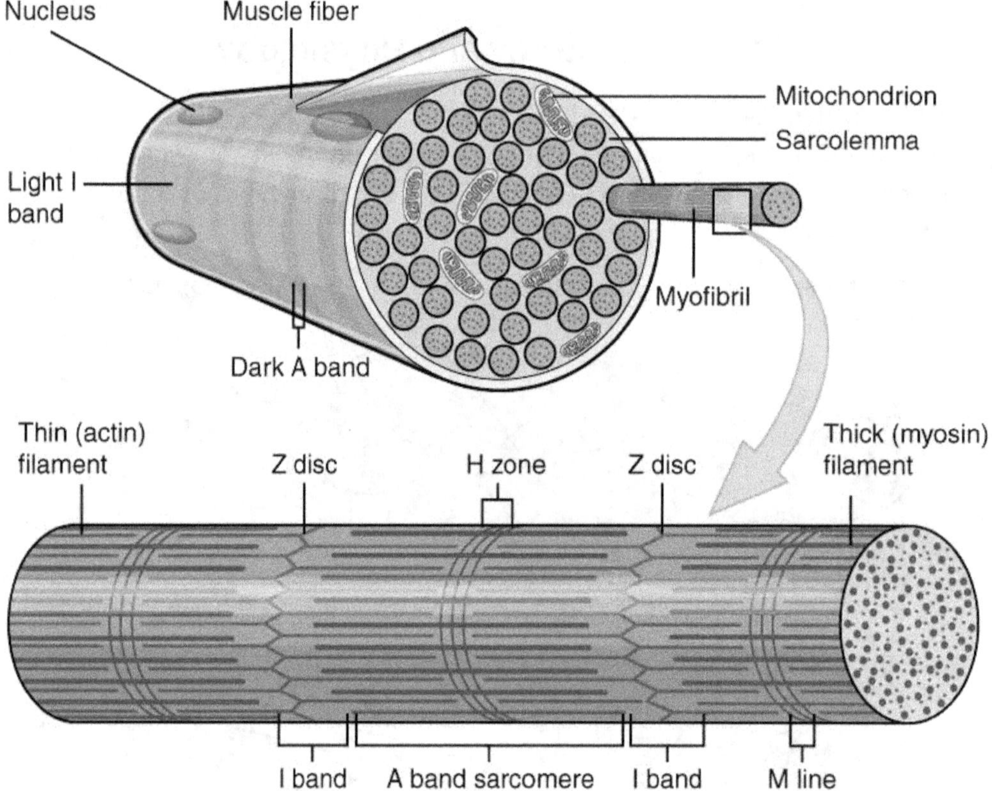

Muscle Actions

- In a **concentric** muscle action, the muscle shortens as it contracts. For example, in the upward phase of a dumbbell bicep curl, the biceps brachii is contracting concentrically to shorten the angle at the elbow and move the dumbbell closer to the body.
- In an **eccentric** muscle action, the muscle lengthens as it contracts. For example, in the descent phase of a squat, the quadriceps muscle group is contracting eccentrically to control the movement.
- In an **isometric** muscle action, the muscle does not change in length during its contraction. For example, when holding a plank, the rectus abdominus contracts isometrically to maintain stability of the trunk.

Most resistance training exercises involve both a concentric and eccentric contraction. Muscle groups work in agonist/antagonist pairs, where one muscle group, the **agonist** (also known as the **prime mover**), is contracting concentrically, and the opposing muscle group, or **antagonist**, is contracting eccentrically. For example, with a bicep curl, the triceps brachii is the antagonist to the biceps brachii and contracts eccentrically on the upward phase. As the biceps brachii contracts eccentrically on the downward phase, the triceps brachii contracts concentrically.

Sliding Filament Theory

The **sliding filament theory** describes the muscular contraction process. During this process, a thin filament (**actin**) slides over a thick filament (**myosin**), which contracts the muscle to generate tension and movement. Calcium is stored in the **sarcoplasmic reticulum**, a network of tubes that surrounds **myofibrils**, which contain the myofilaments actin and myosin. When the sarcoplasmic reticulum is stimulated by an action potential, calcium is released. Calcium then binds with the protein **troponin**, causing another protein, **tropomyosin**, to shift out of the way. This allows actin and myosin to bind by forming cross-bridges. The formation of cross-bridges produces a pulling action, or **power stroke**, which is fueled by the breakdown of ATP. The power stroke from actin and myosin binding shortens muscle fibers, producing muscular contraction through creating tension. The more cross-bridges that are formed between actin and myosin, the greater the force production generated by the muscle.

THE STRETCH-SHORTENING CYCLE

The **stretch-shortening cycle** is a sequence of three events in rapid, powerful muscle contraction where a muscle is quickly stretched and then immediately shortened. The first phase is the **eccentric phase**, where the muscle is stretched by actively lengthening under a load or resistance. This stretching causes the muscles to store elastic energy, like stretching a rubber band. The second phase is called the **amortization phase**. This phase is a brief pause between the eccentric phase and the following concentric phase. A brief amortization phase will result in a more powerful concentric contraction; however, a longer amortization phase will dissipate the previously stored elastic energy, reducing power production in the next phase. The third phase is the **concentric phase**. In this phase, the muscle fibers immediately shorten, causing a rapid muscle contraction. This contraction releases the stored elastic energy from the eccentric phase. The release of stored energy plus the rapid force results in powerful movement.

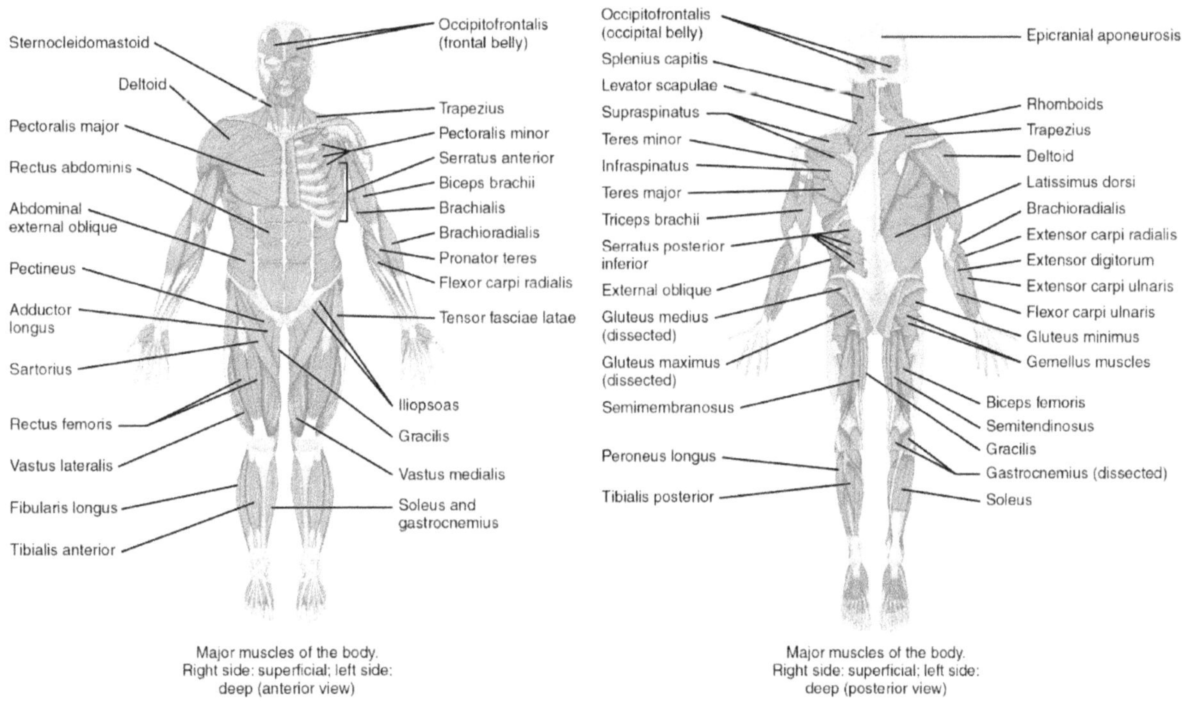

Major muscles of the body. Right side: superficial; left side: deep (anterior view)

Major muscles of the body. Right side: superficial; left side: deep (posterior view)

Muscles That Act on the Hip Joint

- The prime movers involved in hip extension include the gluteus maximus and the hamstrings (biceps femoris, semimembranosus, semitendinosus).
- The prime movers involved in hip flexion include the iliopsoas, rectus femoris, and sartorius.
- The prime movers of hip abduction include the gluteus medius and gluteus minimus.
- The prime movers of hip adduction are the adductor longus, adductor magnus, adductor brevis, pectineus, and gracilis.
- The prime movers in hip external rotation include the piriformis, gluteus maximus, and gemellus muscles.
- Hip internal rotation is not performed by any single prime mover, but muscles that play a role in this movement include the gluteus medius and minimus, tensor fascia latae, adductor longus and brevis, and pectineus.

Muscles That Act on the Glenohumeral Joint and Humerus

- The prime movers in shoulder flexion are the pectoralis major and anterior deltoid.
- The prime movers in shoulder extension are the latissimus dorsi and teres major.
- The prime movers for shoulder abduction are the deltoid (all fibers) and supraspinatus.
- The prime movers for shoulder adduction are the pectoralis major and latissimus dorsi.
- The prime movers for shoulder internal rotation are the latissimus dorsi, pectoralis major, and subscapularis.
- The prime movers for shoulder external rotation are the infraspinatus and teres minor.
- The prime movers for shoulder horizontal abduction are the latissimus dorsi and posterior deltoid.
- The prime movers for shoulder horizontal adduction are the pectoralis major and anterior deltoid.

Muscles That Act on the Knee and Ankle Joints

The knee moves in flexion and extension. Prime movers for knee flexion are the hamstrings (biceps femoris, semimembranosus, semitendinosus). Prime movers for knee extension are the quadriceps (rectus femoris, vastus lateralis, vastus intermedius, vastus medialis).

The ankle moves in plantarflexion, dorsiflexion, eversion, and inversion. Prime movers for ankle plantarflexion (pointing the toes, standing on tiptoes) are the gastrocnemius and soleus. The prime mover for ankle dorsiflexion (pulling the toes closer toward the body) is the anterior tibialis. Prime movers for ankle eversion are the peroneus longus and peroneus brevis. The prime mover for ankle inversion is the anterior tibialis.

Muscles That Act on the Scapula and Elbow

- The prime movers for scapular elevation are the upper trapezius and levator scapulae.
- The prime mover for scapular depression is the lower trapezius.
- The prime movers for scapular adduction (retraction) are the rhomboids and middle trapezius.
- The prime movers for scapular abduction (protraction) are the serratus anterior.
- The prime movers for scapular upward rotation are the upper and middle trapezius.
- The prime movers for scapular downward rotation are the rhomboids.
- The prime movers for elbow flexion are the biceps brachii, brachialis, and brachioradialis.
- The prime mover for elbow extension is the triceps brachii.

- The prime movers for elbow pronation are the pronator teres, pronator quadratus, and flexor carpi radialis.
- The prime movers for elbow supination are the supinator and biceps brachii.

Spinal Movements and Muscles

Spinal flexion is one of the four main spinal movements and involves bending or curving the spine forward, such as when doing a crunch. The prime movers in spinal flexion are the rectus abdominus and the iliopsoas. The opposite of spinal flexion is spinal extension, which involves bending the spine backwards or straightening the spine. The prime movers in extension are the erector spinae group. Lateral spinal flexion, such as in bending to the side, is a third main spinal movement. The prime movers in lateral spinal flexion are the internal obliques, external obliques, and quadratus lumborum. A fourth main spinal movement is rotation, such as in any movement involving twisting from the torso or waist. The internal obliques and external obliques are the prime movers in spinal rotation. More specifically, the ipsilateral (same side) internal oblique and the contralateral (opposite side) external oblique are active. For example, rotating to the right involves the prime movers of the internal oblique on the right side and the external oblique on the left side.

Neuromuscular Anatomy and Physiology

Motor Units

The **motor unit** is the functional unit of the neuromuscular system. Motor units are located in the space between muscle fibers and motor neurons, which is called the **neuromuscular junction**. The role the motor unit in muscle contraction starts when it is stimulated by the motor neuron. Then, the motor unit provokes muscle fibers to contract. The role of motor units in muscle contraction follows the **all-or-none principle**, where all muscle fibers of a given motor unit simultaneously contract. Additionally, all motor units in a muscle must be activated to produce maximal force.

All motor units innervate muscle fibers but not necessarily the same number of muscle fibers. Depending on the muscle, a given motor unit may innervate hundreds of fibers or just a single fiber. Motor units in muscles that contract with high force but low precision, such as the gluteals, quadriceps, or hamstrings, have a ratio of one motor neuron to many muscle fibers. Conversely, motor units in muscles that contract with low force but higher precision, such as the small muscles in the eyeball or fingers, have a ratio of one motor neuron to just a few muscle fibers.

Type I and Type II Muscle Fibers

Type I (**slow-twitch**) muscle fibers develop force slowly over a longer period of time and have a high aerobic capacity. Their aerobic properties are due to multiple factors, such as having more capillaries that allow increased oxygen transport, and having more **mitochondria**, which generate energy through aerobic metabolism. Because of their slower and longer duration of force development and high aerobic capacity, Type I muscle fibers are more resistant to fatigue and best suited to muscular endurance.

In contrast, **type II** (**fast-twitch**) muscle fibers are characterized by rapid force development in a short period of time. They do not have a high aerobic capacity, as the number of capillaries and mitochondria in type II fibers is low, so they have a lower blood supply and contain less oxygen; however, their anaerobic capacity is high due to generating energy through anaerobic metabolism, where large amounts of **myosin ATPase** break down ATP as a quick, short-lasting source of energy. They are best suited for high power output because they contract quickly and conduct nerve impulses quickly, though they are less fatigue-resistant since these high intensities cannot be sustained for extended periods.

Muscle Spindles

Muscle spindles are **proprioceptors** that sense the length of a muscle (i.e., its level of tension relative to its normal resting length) and the rate of change in muscle length. They are located within specialized muscle fibers and have sensory neurons that detect the properties of the muscle when it is stretched. Muscle spindles use these sensory neurons to send their signals to the spinal cord, which then sends motor signals back to the muscle to control its contraction. Based on a given resistance, the muscle spindle signals how strongly the muscle must be activated. A greater resistance means more muscle activation from a higher engagement of muscle spindles. For example, a rapid stretch of a muscle will cause the muscle spindles to increase the contractile activity in the muscle.

Golgi Tendon Organs

Golgi tendon organs (GTOs) are **proprioceptors** that activate when a muscle's tendon is stretched. They are located at each end of a muscle within the tendons that serve as the muscle's attachment to bone. Golgi tendon organs have sensory neurons to detect muscle tension. When a muscle is stretched, the GTO's signal to the spinal cord inhibits motor neurons in the muscle, which also inhibits muscular activation, causing the muscle to relax. The role of the GTO can be conceptualized as the opposite of the muscle spindle, where GTO activation reduces muscle tension and promotes muscle relaxation, compared to muscle spindle activation that promotes muscular contraction.

Motor Unit Recruitment Patterns

Motor unit recruitment is the process by which motor neurons activate muscle fibers to produce movement. Their pattern of activation typically follows the **size principle**, where motor neurons with smaller motor units are recruited first, followed by motor neurons with larger motor units. This is because smaller motor units produce less force, so they can be recruited first without causing the muscle to contract too forcefully. As the force, speed, or power required for the movement increases, larger motor units are recruited to meet the demands of the movement; however, in high-speed, explosive movements, **selective recruitment** is possible, where larger motor units are recruited first to provide the greatest force production.

Nerve Conduction

The path of nerve conduction involves electrical signals traveling through the nervous system to reach muscles. Nerve conduction begins when an **action potential** is generated in a motor neuron. The action potential is like an electric current traveling down the axon of the motor neuron. The axon acts as wiring to transmit the current. The destination for the action potential is the neuromuscular junction. Reaching this destination causes the release of **acetylcholine**, a neurotransmitter that produces an excitatory response in the **sarcolemma**, the cell membrane surrounding each muscle fiber. This excitatory response is responsible for muscle contraction. The speed of nerve conduction is different based on muscle fiber type. Type II muscle fibers have fast nerve conduction velocities, and type I muscle fibers have slower nerve conduction velocities.

Twitch, Summation, and Tetanus

Twitch, summation (also known as twitch summation), and tetanus can be thought of as muscle contraction force from smallest to largest. A **twitch** is where muscle fibers briefly contract as a result of a single action potential that travels from a motor neuron. This brief contraction does not have a large amount of force. In **summation**, multiple twitches overlap and produce a greater contractile force compared to a single twitch. This can occur when multiple action potentials are generated in rapid succession or when a single action potential is prolonged. **Tetanus** is the maximal amount of force possible from an action potential. Tetanus occurs when multiple action potentials are generated at a very rapid rate, creating successive twitches that merge to create a combined high level of force.

Basic Principles of Biomechanics

Anatomical Planes

The three anatomical planes divide the body into sections, which can be thought of as three imaginary lines that slice through the body and intersect at the center.

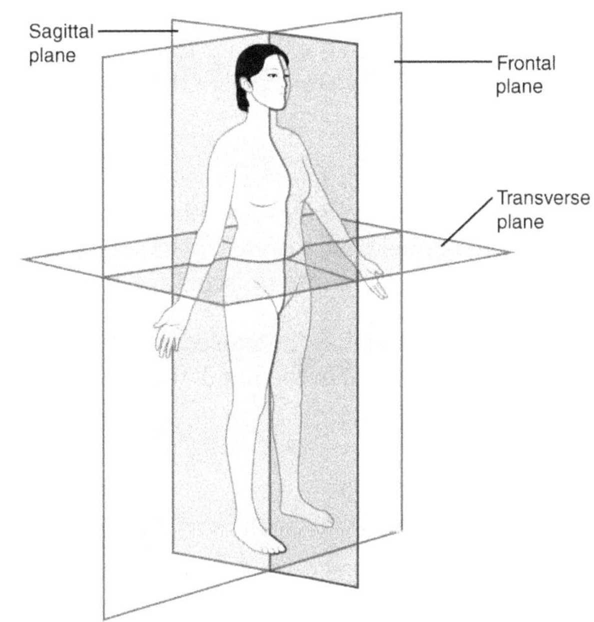

The **sagittal plane** divides the body into right and left halves. **Sagittal plane movements** are any movements that occur parallel to this line. For example, forward lunges and bicep curls are sagittal plane movements.

The **frontal plane** divides the body into front and back halves. **Frontal plane movements** are any movements that occur parallel to this dividing line, such as movements that are lateral (to the right or left side). For example, side shuffles and lateral raises are frontal plane movements.

The **transverse plane** divides the body into superior and inferior, or upper and lower halves, with the imaginary line typically conceptualized at waistline level. **Transverse plane movements** are any movements parallel to this line, such as rotational movements. For example, golf swings and baseball pitches are transverse plane movements.

Joint Angle

The force a muscle can produce depends on its length, which is determined by the joint angle. The **joint angle** is the angle between two bones that are connected by a joint. For example, the joint angle for the knee is determined by the angle between the femur and the tibia.

When the joint angle is small, the muscle can produce more force. Conversely, when the joint angle is larger, the muscle's force-producing ability decreases. Imagine someone who is about to perform a vertical jump. They will bend at the knees before jumping (shortening the joint angle at the knee) to produce a higher amount of force than jumping with nearly straight legs, which has a large joint angle at the knee.

Force-Velocity Relationship

Velocity is the speed of a muscle's change in length. During muscular contraction, a rapid change in length happens at a high velocity, and a slower change in length happens at a lower velocity.

There is an inverse relationship between force and velocity in muscle contraction. A movement that requires near-maximal amounts of force, such as a 1-repetition maximum (1-RM) deadlift, does not occur at high velocity. Conversely, higher velocity changes in muscle can only be accomplished with much lighter loading on the muscle, reducing the force it needs to generate.

Power is the product of force and velocity. The power of muscular contractions can be improved through training either at higher forces (such as heavier loads of weight) or higher velocities (such as more explosive speed of movement). Most athletic activities will benefit from a range of forces and velocities in training to optimize power across different movement demands.

Levers

There are three basic types of levers that act to pull on bones in muscular contractions. Each lever has muscular force, resistive force, and an axis. The **axis**, also known as the **fulcrum**, is at the center of a joint, and the muscles crossing that joint act as the levers.

A **first-class lever** has the axis point between the muscular force and the resistive force. The joint attaching the skull to the first vertebra is a first-class lever. The muscular force is from the neck muscles that attach to the back of the skull, the resistive force is the weight of the skull, and the axis is between them.

A **second-class lever** has the resistive force between the axis and the muscular force. Standing on the tips of the toes involves dorsiflexion using the joints at the toes. The muscular force for this movement comes from the gastrocnemius and soleus muscles, and the resistive force of gravity acts downward between those muscles and the joints of the toes (the axis).

A **third-class lever** has the muscular force between the axis and the resistive force. In a bicep curl, the resistance is held in the hand, the axis is the elbow joint, and the muscular force from the biceps is between them.

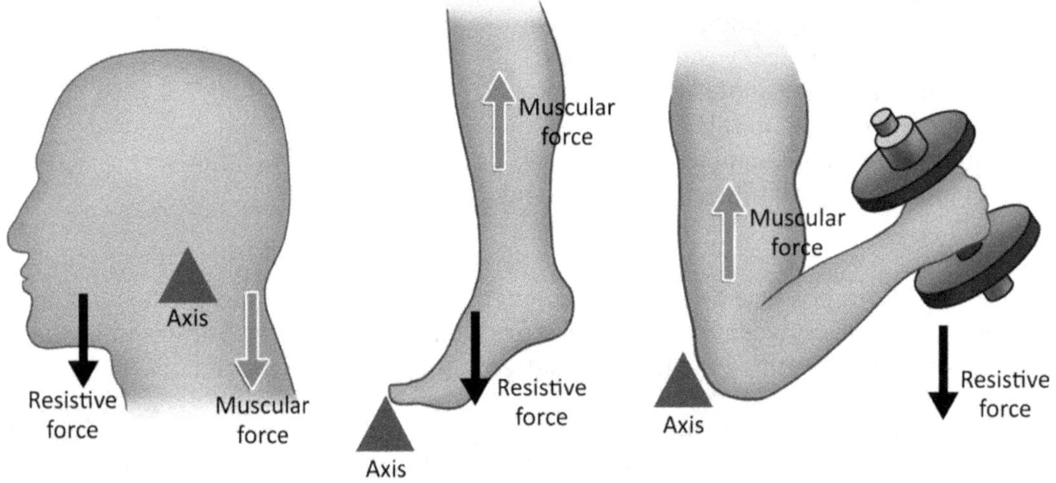

Torque and Moment Arm

In muscular contraction, **torque** is the turning force applied relative to a joint angle. The **moment arm** is the perpendicular distance from the point of rotation to the line of action of the force. In relation to muscular contraction, the moment arm of the force exerted on bones by muscle fibers is the distance from the joint to the point of muscle attachment. Because gravity is a constant vertical force that acts on the human body, the moment arm runs horizontally (perpendicular to gravity's vertical force). The greater the moment arm, the more torque that is exerted on the joint and the more force required to counteract gravity.

For example, in a dumbbell front raise, the force of the deltoids contracting creates torque that allows the weight to be lifted and counteract gravity's vertical force. The moment arm of this force is the distance from the shoulder joint to the line of action of gravitational force. Therefore, a front raise will require the most torque when the moment arm is the longest, which is when the arms are horizontal and the dumbbells are the furthest from the body.

Agonists, Antagonists, and Synergists

Muscles typically do not work in isolation in muscular contraction but have assistance from other muscles to counteract and assist the forces they produce. An **agonist**, also called the prime mover, is the muscle most responsible for a movement. An **antagonist** is a muscle that works in opposition to the agonist by slowing down the agonist's movement to control the speed of muscular contraction. A **synergist** is a muscle that provides indirect assistance to an agonist but is not the prime mover.

For example, in a bench press, the agonists for the pushing motion are the pectoralis major muscles. The antagonist muscles are the latissimus dorsi muscles. The anterior deltoids and triceps brachii muscles function as synergists to assist the pectoralis major.

Neutralizers and Stabilizers

Neutralizers provide counteracting forces to the agonist muscles and/or the assisting synergist muscles in a movement. Neutralizers are different from antagonists because antagonists work directly in opposition, but neutralizers moderate or reduce unwanted joint movement by the agonist or synergists. Movements with hip extension are a good example to illustrate the role of neutralizers. The gluteus maximus is the agonist in hip extension and is also the agonist for hip external rotation. During hip extension, the gluteus minimus, hip internal rotators, and tensor fascia latae function as neutralizers to counteract hip external rotation.

Stabilizers maintain the positions of bones during agonist contraction. The postural muscles, such as spinal muscles, transverse abdominus, and rectus abdominus, are recruited as stabilizers in most types of multi-joint or compound movements. For example, in a back squat, these muscles stabilize the position of the spine and pelvis, allowing the agonist muscles in the legs to exert more force.

Bone and Connective Tissue Anatomy and Physiology

Bone Anatomy

Trabecular bone (also known as spongy bone) is the tissue within a bone that contains bone marrow. This is where blood cells are produced. The hard outer covering of a bone is called **cortical bone** (also known as compact bone). The outermost membrane surrounding the bone is called the **periosteum**. Tendon attachment connects skeletal muscles to the periosteum to enable muscles to pull on bones. The periosteum is the primary site for new bone formation. **Osteoblasts** are cells that build new bone on the periosteum by depositing collagen proteins that eventually form bone. **Subchondral tissue** is located at the ends of a bone and is covered with **cartilage**, a type of connective tissue that absorbs forces on bones and provides a smooth surface for movement.

Tendons, Ligaments, and Fascia

Tendons, ligaments, and fascia are all types of connective tissue with specific roles in muscular contraction. They are made of **collagen fibers**, which are made from protein. Like how muscle fibers are arranged in bundles to form a muscle, collagen fibers in longitudinal parallel bundles form tendons and ligaments. Fascia is formed by sheets of collagen arranged in multidirectional bundles like a network of mesh or a web. Fascia holds muscles together.

Tendons attach muscles to bones, and **ligaments** attach one bone to another. Both tendons and ligaments function to transmit force to bones during muscle contraction. **Fascia** helps absorb and transmit forces. Tendons and ligaments do not connect to each other in the body, but tendons and fascia are connected. The fascia that covers a muscle forms the muscle tendon at the end of the muscle.

Types of Joints

There are three main types of joints involved in muscle contraction. Joints can be classified based on the amount of movement around their axes of rotation.

Uniaxial joints have one axis of rotation and move only in one plane of motion. These are also known as hinge joints because their movement is limited to flexion and extension or opening and closing like a hinge. Uniaxial joints have the highest levels of stability compared to the other two types. The elbow and knee are examples of uniaxial joints.

Biaxial joints have two axes of rotation and can move in two planes of motion. For example, the ankle and wrist can flex and extend as well as move laterally.

Multiaxial joints, also termed **ball-and-socket joints,** have three axes of rotation and can move in all three planes of motion. The shoulder and the hip are examples of multiaxial joints, as they can flex, extend, move laterally, internally and externally rotate, and perform circumduction. Multiaxial joints have the most freedom of movement compared to the other two types.

Bone Remodeling in Response to Mechanical Loading

Mechanical loading, such as through weight-bearing exercise and training, places stress on bones. An appropriate amount of stress that is not excessive stimulates osteoblasts to produce collagen proteins. This threshold of stress is called the **minimal essential strain (MES)**. This occurs when there is an overload beyond normal resting levels. The collagen proteins become part of the bone's outer surface, increasing **bone mineral density** and strength.

Wolff's law dictates that bones adapt and remodel along the lines of stresses that are placed on them. For example, bones subjected to repeated loading will remodel, becoming stronger to withstand that loading. Conversely, bones that are not loaded beyond the minimal essential strain will not receive adequate stress to adapt and remodel. The greatest extent of bone adaptation occurs in full-body, multi-joint movements that load the axial skeleton (the spine). These types of movements use large muscle groups, providing more stimulus to bones than isolated, single-joint movements.

Tendon and Ligament Remodeling in Response to Mechanical Loading

Since tendons attach bones to muscles and ligaments join bones together, the main adaptations in response to mechanical loading come from stresses placed on the skeletal system and muscular system. For example, the forces generated by muscle contraction provoke greater pulling force in tendons and ligaments. If this loading stress is within the amount of load that these connective tissues can withstand, the tendons or ligaments will increase in strength and their capacity to transmit force. These adaptations are from changes in the collagen fibers that make up tendons and ligaments, such as an increased number of collagen fibers, increased size of collagen fibers, and the production of more densely packed collagen fibers. High-intensity exercise creates a higher degree of tissue adaptations in response to loading than lower intensity exercise.

Muscle Adaptations to Training

Muscle adaptations in the first few weeks of training are not due to physical changes in the muscle but from improved neural adaptations in muscle contraction, such as the ability to recruit more motor units or a faster firing rate of the motor units. As training continues, muscles can increase in size (termed **hypertrophy**) due to an increased cross-sectional area of muscle fibers. This is due to increased amounts of actin and myosin proteins and an increased number of myofibrils. Having more of these components also allows muscles to generate more force. The repeated contraction of muscle fibers, such as through training, also stimulates pathways that increase **myogenesis**, or muscle growth and protein synthesis. The principle of **specificity** dictates what other adaptations will occur based on the nature of training. For example, training for endurance makes muscles adapt to being more fatigue-resistant, and training for power makes muscles adapt to generating more force rapidly.

Bioenergetics and Metabolism

Anaerobic and Aerobic Metabolism

In the context of biological energy systems, **metabolism** encompasses all reactions where energy is released or stored. This includes breaking down macronutrients into smaller molecules (e.g., breaking carbohydrates down to form ATP), or building complex molecules from smaller ones (e.g., synthesizing protein from amino acids).

Anaerobic metabolism occurs in the absence of oxygen and includes the phosphagen system and glycolytic system. Anaerobic metabolism occurs in the sarcoplasm of muscle cells and uses carbohydrates as its main macronutrient energy source, as carbohydrates do not require oxygen to be broken down to use as energy for the body.

Aerobic metabolism requires oxygen and includes the Krebs cycle, electron transport system, and oxidative system. Aerobic metabolism occurs in the mitochondria and can use all three macronutrients—fats, carbohydrates, and proteins—as energy sources.

Both anaerobic and aerobic metabolism—and their corresponding systems—are always active in the body; however, aerobic metabolism is more active during longer-duration, lower-intensity activity, while anaerobic metabolism is more active during short-duration, higher-intensity activity.

Phosphagen System

The **phosphagen system** is both the most immediate and the fastest energy system. It is active at the start of all activity and is the primary system during extremely high-intensity, short term muscle contraction, such as a maximal lift or a few seconds of all-out sprinting.

The phosphagen system derives its energy from breaking down **phosphocreatine (PCr)**, also termed **creatine phosphate (CP)**. When combined with ADP (adenosine diphosphate), the enzyme **creatine kinase** provides the catalyst for creatine phosphate and ADP to synthesize ATP, allowing the transfer of energy for muscle contraction.

A limiting factor of the phosphagen system is that it cannot be used as the primary energy source of ATP beyond short durations. This is because only small amounts of creatine phosphate are stored in the body, hence why someone cannot exercise at a maximal effort for more than a few seconds.

Glycolytic System

The **glycolytic system** is so named because it derives its energy from **glycolysis**, which is the breakdown of carbohydrates. This breakdown of carbohydrates results in **pyruvate**, an acid that can either be used for anaerobic or aerobic metabolism depending on where it goes next, which is based on the energy demands of the activity.

Conversion of pyruvate to lactate allows rapid synthesis of ATP, termed **anaerobic glycolysis** or **fast glycolysis.** Anaerobic glycolysis is used as the primary energy system in moderately high to very high intensity activity lasting anywhere from more than a few seconds up to a few minutes. Anaerobic glycolysis is less rapid and immediate than the phosphagen system.

If pyruvate goes into the mitochondria, it undergoes the **Krebs cycle**, also known as the **citric acid cycle**, which allows ATP to be synthesized at a slower rate that lasts for a longer duration. This is termed **aerobic glycolysis**, or **slow glycolysis.** Aerobic glycolysis is used as an energy system in lower intensity, longer duration activities.

Oxidative System

The **oxidative system** only functions in the presence of oxygen and is the main energy system for aerobic metabolism, which works during activities that are lower in intensity and that last longer than around 3 minutes. Compared to the systems in anaerobic metabolism, which only use carbohydrates for fuel, the oxidative system can derive energy from all three macronutrients (carbohydrates, fats, and protein), with carbohydrates and fats as the primary sources. Metabolic reactions in the mitochondria can break macronutrients down into large amounts of ATP but at a slower rate than the systems in anaerobic metabolism.

Carbohydrates used in aerobic metabolism come from blood glucose and muscle glycogen, which are broken down through **glycolysis** and then enter the Krebs cycle in the mitochondria. ATP is the end result, produced through what is termed **oxidative phosphorylation**. Fats used in aerobic metabolism come from triglycerides broken down into free fatty acids, which enter the mitochondria and undergo **beta oxidation**. Fat as an energy source supplies the greatest amount of ATP molecules. Protein in aerobic metabolism can undergo **gluconeogenesis** to convert to glucose or enter the Krebs cycle to become ATP.

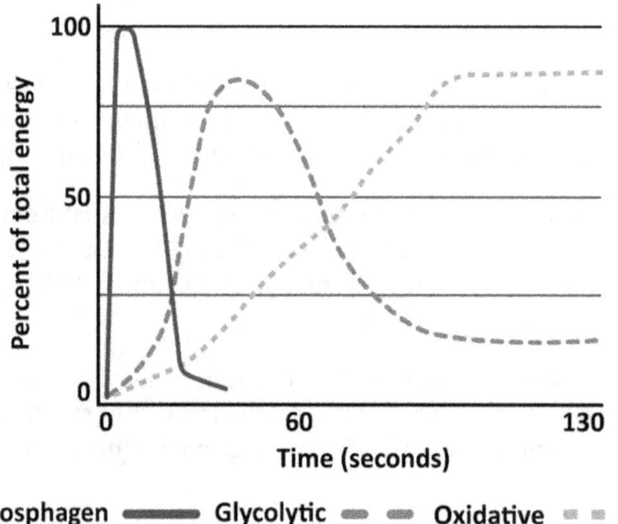

Manipulation of Training Variables to Target Energy Systems

According to the **principle of specificity**, improving the function and efficiency of each energy system will require modulating training variables targeted to that energy system's use. These training variables may include intensity and recovery time.

Since the phosphagen system and glycolytic system are most active within the first minute of activity, effective training for these systems involves short bursts of intense or near-maximal activity. This type of training can also improve the concentration of stored muscle glycogen. The more intense or maximal the activity, the longer the recovery time should be to allow anaerobic energy stores to be replenished. For example, an all-out burst of intensity for 5–10 seconds warrants a rest period of 2 minutes or more.

Effectively training the oxidative system focuses on maximizing aerobic metabolism pathways through longer duration and lower intensity activity with shorter recovery times. This builds the body's efficiency at supplying energy using oxygen, such as increasing oxygen uptake over time.

Oxygen Uptake, Oxygen Deficit, and Oxygen Debt

Oxygen uptake refers to how effectively the body can take in oxygen and deliver it to the heart, lungs, and muscles. An individual's maximal oxygen uptake is measured as VO_2 max. This represents the highest achievable maximal exercise intensity and is also known as maximal aerobic capacity. Oxygen uptake can be improved through training that focuses primarily on aerobic metabolism.

Anaerobic metabolism provides energy at the start of exercise (for about the first minute) with its faster rate of ATP synthesis. Anaerobic metabolism's contribution of energy is termed the **oxygen deficit** since it does not use oxygen. The slower-responding, longer-lasting aerobic metabolism takes over as the primary energy pathway after about a minute of exercise.

Oxygen debt, also known as **excess post-exercise oxygen consumption (EPOC)**, is the amount of oxygen the body needs to restore homeostasis after finishing exercise. EPOC is most influenced by intensity, where high-intensity exercise produces longer EPOC phases than lower intensity exercise.

The Lactate Threshold

Lactate is a byproduct of pyruvate and is produced during anaerobic metabolism. There is a linear relationship between exercise intensity and blood lactate concentration where more intense levels of exercise increase lactate production. The **lactate threshold** is the exercise intensity where blood lactate concentration rapidly increases above baseline levels. This point also typically represents the **anaerobic threshold**, where anaerobic metabolism provides a significant contribution because the intensity is too high for the body to rely on aerobic metabolism alone.

Training adaptations can reduce lactate production and enable the body to buffer or clear lactate more efficiently. This means that a trained individual can exercise at a percentage of their maximal oxygen uptake (VO_2 max) before meeting the lactate threshold.

Using Interval Training to Train Specific Energy Systems

Interval training uses work periods and recovery periods at predetermined ratios to train specific energy systems. Interval training can be used to improve the efficiency of either anaerobic or aerobic metabolism depending on the **work-to-rest ratio**. For example, since aerobic metabolism is most active in lower intensity training that lasts 3 minutes or longer, interval training for aerobic metabolism might involve repeated bouts of 3–5 minutes of submaximal work with an equal amount of rest or active recovery. Since training that relies on anaerobic metabolism can only be sustained for short periods, interval training allows anaerobic metabolism to be utilized in repeated, intense bouts followed by recovery where the body can replenish its fuel stores.

High-intensity interval training (HIIT) is a specific type of interval training where the work periods are brief but very intense (about 90% of VO_2 max). This type of training not only improves anaerobic metabolism, such as by increasing the anaerobic threshold and creating muscle fiber adaptations, but it is also a time-efficient way to improve VO_2 max without doing long durations of submaximal intensity training.

Neuroendocrine Physiology

Types of Hormones

Hormones can be divided into three categories based on their molecular structures. **Steroid hormones** come from the reproductive glands and the adrenal cortex. Testosterone, estrogen, and cortisol are steroidal hormones. **Polypeptide** (also known as **peptide**) **hormones** come from specialized cells throughout the body and are composed of amino acid chains. They include insulin and growth hormone. **Amine hormones** are derived from amino acids. They include **catecholamines**, which are hormones that also act as neurotransmitters to send signals in the body's stress response, such as epinephrine (adrenaline), norepinephrine, and dopamine.

Among the many hormones that have potential involvement in exercise, the most prominent are the catecholamines, which act in the body's acute **fight-or-flight** stress response to exercise. This response is enacted by the sympathetic nervous system in response to stress. Effects such as increased heart rate and increased muscle tension are associated with this stress response. Catecholamines enhance the action of the vascular system and muscles in exercise, resulting in effects like improved blood flow to muscles and improved muscle force production.

Hormones Related to Exercise

Hormones are chemical messengers of the endocrine system that bind to specific receptor sites. Hormones are released by **endocrine glands**, such as the hypothalamus, adrenal glands, kidneys, reproductive glands, and other sites in the body.

Hormones interact with cells in the body to provide three basic functions. **Anabolic hormones** require energy and promote the building of new tissue, such as building new muscle. **Permissive hormones** allow other hormones to act by functioning as precursors to maximize hormonal effects. **Catabolic hormones** release energy through breaking down molecules, such as breaking down muscle glycogen to be used as fuel if the body needs it.

In general, exercise provides a stimulus for hormonal interactions to occur beyond daily hormonal maintenance of homeostasis. For example, exercise elevates some anabolic hormones, promoting protein synthesis and muscle growth; however, excessive stress on the body, like from overtraining, can elevate catabolic hormones and impair muscle recovery.

Cortisol

Cortisol, a steroid hormone produced by the adrenal cortex, naturally fluctuates throughout the day and has different effects on the body depending on homeostatic needs. For example, cortisol rises if muscle glycogen levels are low. It may also rise in response to intense or high-volume exercise. Such a rise in cortisol prompts catabolic reactions in the body, such as metabolizing carbohydrates and breaking down proteins to keep muscles fueled. Therefore, an acute rise in cortisol in response to exercise is not automatically negative, as it can continue to fuel exercise and provoke positive adaptations over time.

Prolonged periods of elevated cortisol, however, reduce the extent of the body's adaptations to exercise. Such prolonged periods of elevated cortisol may arise when an athlete is not recovering adequately from exercise or not refueling their muscle glycogen through proper nutrition. In these cases, cortisol works to conserve fuel, such as by using amino acids rather than having them undergo protein synthesis or by catabolizing muscle protein. Overall, the effects of cortisol emphasize the importance of balancing exercise and recovery to maximize exercise adaptations.

TESTOSTERONE

Testosterone is a steroid hormone that is produced by the adrenal glands and reproductive glands (testes in males and ovaries in females). Testosterone's function is anabolic, and it is one of the main hormones responsible for building muscle tissue. More specifically, testosterone can work synergistically with other hormones—such as growth hormone—to promote protein synthesis. Testosterone can also bind with specific receptors and interact with neurotransmitters to increase muscle mass and force production.

Testosterone levels fluctuate throughout the day in both sexes; however, males have much higher circulating testosterone levels than females and, therefore, typically have more muscle mass and higher strength levels. Testosterone levels increase in response to exercise, and specific exercise variables like volume and intensity can be manipulated to elicit further increases.

GROWTH HORMONE

Growth hormone has multiple variants within the body and is influenced by a variety of factors, but it generally contributes to resistance training adaptations. It is secreted by the anterior pituitary gland and is an anabolic hormone that promotes muscle growth. Some of growth hormone's other effects related to exercise training adaptations include increased protein synthesis, increased collagen synthesis for muscle repair, and promoting the breakdown and use of fat as fuel.

Growth hormone is partially mediated by another hormone, **insulin-like growth factor 1 (IGF-1)**, an anabolic hormone produced in the liver. Both growth hormone and IGF-1 may increase in response to intense resistance training due to the overloading of muscle cells. These two hormones also play a role in promoting muscle tissue repair in response to exercise stressors.

TRAINING MANIPULATIONS TO MAXIMIZE THE EFFECTS OF ADRENAL HORMONES

The main adrenal hormones relevant to exercise and recovery are the **catecholamines** (specifically, epinephrine and norepinephrine) and cortisol. An appropriate exercise stimulus provokes an acute **stress response**, raising catecholamine levels and mobilizing the body to handle the stress through increasing physiological processes like breaking down energy for use and increasing muscle force and contraction. With training, the body can adapt to higher levels of catecholamine secretion. Variables in optimizing this response to training include using compound exercises with large muscle groups, high volume and/or high intensity, and short rest periods.

Appropriate recovery is just as important as the training stimuli, however. Periodization should include full rest days and varied rest periods, intensities, and volumes. This will aid in recovery and help avoid overtaxing the adrenal glands through the chronic release of cortisol. Excessive adrenal activity and chronically elevated levels of cortisol can delay recovery, impair catecholamine release, and lead to overtraining.

Increasing Anabolic Hormones through Training

Anabolic hormones, such as testosterone, growth hormone, and IGF-1 are instrumental in making training gains since they are the primary hormones involved in muscle growth and repair. Training for muscle growth and remodeling—and therefore maximizing the effects of anabolic hormones—necessitates maximizing the amount of muscle fibers used. Exercise choices for increasing anabolic hormones include compound exercises with large muscle groups that are done at high intensities or against heavy resistance, such as a 10-rep maximum set or repetitions at 85–95% of the person's 1-rep max. The training stimulus should also involve high volume with multiple exercises or multiple sets (at least 3). In addition, rest periods should be kept short at 1–2 minutes. Consuming carbohydrates and protein before and after a workout can also enhance the body's concentration of IGF-1.

Cardiopulmonary Anatomy and Physiology

Structures of the Heart

The heart consists of four chambers. The upper chambers are the right and left **atria**, and the lower chambers are the right and left **ventricles**. The atria act as receiving chambers for blood and contract to push blood into the ventricles, while the ventricles serve as the primary pumping chambers of the heart. **Systole** is the contraction of the ventricles, and **diastole** is the relaxation of the ventricles.

The valves of the heart keep blood flowing in one direction, like one-way doors. The valves between the atria and ventricles are called the **atrioventricular valves**. The valve on the right is the **tricuspid valve**, and the valve on the left is the **bicuspid valve**. These atrioventricular valves prevent backflow of blood into the atria when the ventricles contract during systole. At the base of each ventricle are the **semilunar valves**. These valves prevent backflow of blood into the ventricles when they are relaxing during diastole.

Electrical Conduction System of the Heart

The heart's specialized cardiac muscle, or **myocardium,** has cells with their own conduction systems, which enables them to generate power without conscious control, unlike skeletal muscle. The normal rhythm of the heart is established by the **sinoatrial (SA) node**, known as the pacemaker of the heart, which is located in the upper right atrium. Electrical impulses generated in the SA node travel through internodal pathways to the **atrioventricular (AV) node** and then pass through the **atrioventricular (AV) bundle** to make their way to the ventricles. Within the ventricles, the **left** and **right bundle branches** receive the impulse, transmitting it to both ventricles simultaneously through the **Purkinje fibers**. The heart receives input on rhythm from the **parasympathetic** and **sympathetic nervous system** as part of the **autonomic nervous system**. Increased parasympathetic activity produces slowing of the heart rate, while increased sympathetic activity produces increased heart rate.

Systemic Circulation

The **arterial system** transports blood away from the heart to the rest of the body. This begins with oxygen-depleted blood entering the right atrium of the heart through the **superior vena cava** and **inferior vena cava**. Next, blood flows through the **tricuspid valve** into the right ventricle, which pumps the blood into the lungs through **pulmonary arteries**. In the lungs, the blood receives oxygen and disposes of carbon dioxide. The oxygen-rich blood returns to the left atrium of the heart through **pulmonary veins** and flows into the left ventricle via the **mitral valve**. The left ventricle then pumps the blood into the rest of the body through the **aortic valve** and then the **aorta.** Blood travels successively through **arteries**, **arterioles**, and then to **capillaries**, where nutrient and gas exchange occurs.

The **venous system** returns blood back to the heart. Blood from the capillaries goes through **venules** and then **veins** to be transported back to the right ventricle, which pumps oxygen-poor blood into the lungs. The lungs replenish oxygen in the blood, and the blood travels to the left atrium of the heart.

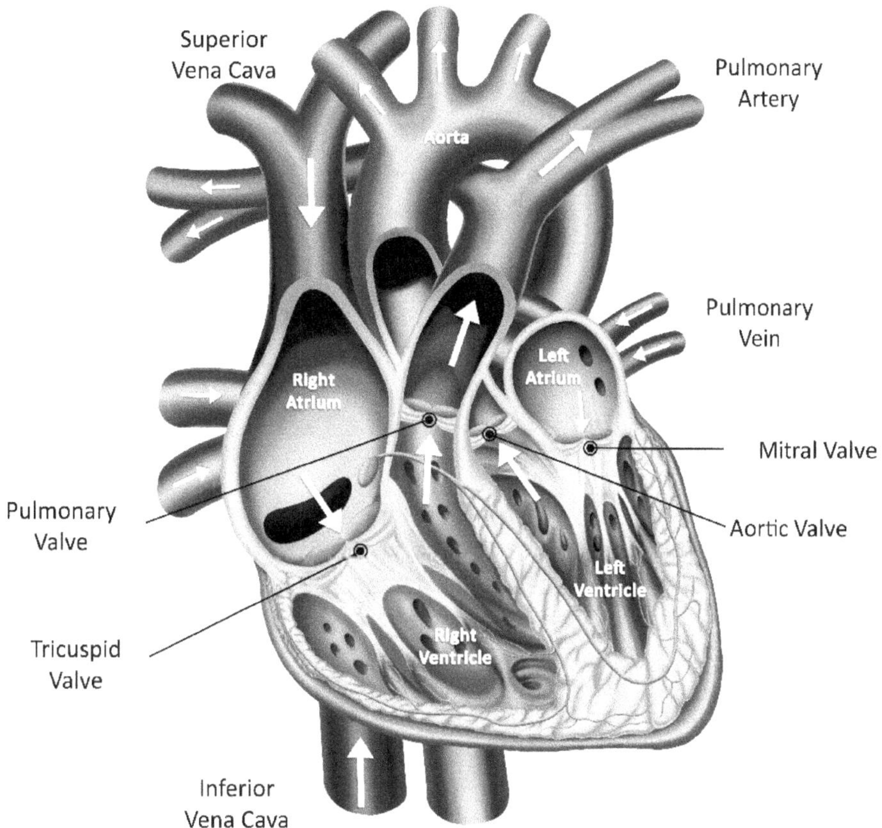

Respiratory System

The **respiratory system** takes in oxygen to use as fuel and expels carbon dioxide as a waste product. Air is inhaled through the nose and passes through the nasal cavities. The air then travels through passages of the respiratory system that branch off into progressively smaller components. The first passage is the **trachea**, which divides into right and left **bronchi**, one for each lung. The bronchi branch off further into smaller passages called **bronchioles**. The next destination for inhaled air is the **alveoli**, where gas exchange occurs. The alveoli have capillary membranes that allow **diffusion**, where oxygen enters the blood and carbon dioxide is removed from the blood.

The **diaphragm** is the main muscle involved in breathing. During inhalation, its contraction creates a vacuum that draws air into the lungs, and during exhalation, it relaxes to allow expelling air. When breathing demands are greater, such as during exercise, other muscles act as synergists. **Muscles of inspiration** (external intercostals, sternocleidomastoids, anterior serratus, scalenes) elevate the rib cage to further expand the lungs. **Muscles of expiration** (abdominal muscles, internal intercostals) depress the chest and allow more forceful exhalation.

The Respiratory System

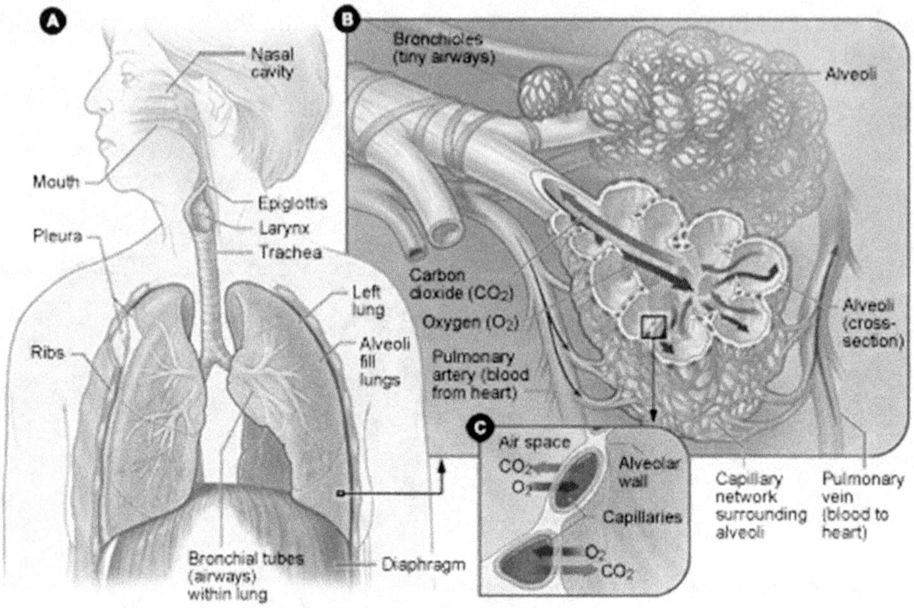

Cardiac Responses to Training

Heart rate, or the rate of pumping per minute, responds linearly to the intensity of exercise. **Maximal heart rate (MHR)** is the highest estimated heart rate at which an individual can exercise. MHR is often calculated as 220 minus the person's age, but this is only a general estimate because heart rate responses depend on a variety of factors.

Stroke volume is the amount of blood the heart ejects with each beat (typically measured in milliliters). In acute response to exercise, stroke volume rises until about 40–50% of VO_2 max and then levels off. Increased stroke volume as an acute response to exercise occurs for two reasons—more blood is returning to the heart to match the demands of exercise, and the sympathetic nervous system induces the ventricles and venous system to contract more forcefully.

Cardiac output is the product of heart rate and stroke volume and is the quantity of blood pumped by the heart (typically measured in liters per minute). Cardiac output has a rapid acute response to exercise before reaching a gradual increase and then leveling off.

Blood pressure has two components. **Systolic blood pressure** is when the heart's ventricles contract to eject blood, and **diastolic blood pressure** is when the ventricles relax. Systolic blood pressure has a linear increase with exercise intensity, while diastolic pressure will remain the same as it was at resting levels or slightly decrease.

Respiratory Responses to Training

The body constantly needs oxygen for fuel, and **oxygen uptake (VO_2)** is the amount consumed. The average estimated amount of oxygen uptake for an individual at rest is 3.5 milliliters per kilogram of body weight per minute, which is termed one **metabolic equivalent (MET)**. In acute response to exercise, oxygen uptake increases because the working muscles require more oxygen than when at rest. This increase is a linear response based on intensity. An individual's highest oxygen uptake, representing the highest intensity their cardiopulmonary system can reach, is termed **VO_2 max**, or **maximal oxygen uptake**.

Minute ventilation is the amount of air breathed each minute. **Tidal volume** is the amount of air inhaled and exhaled per breath. Ventilation increases in response to exercise, since more oxygen is consumed and more carbon dioxide is produced compared to being at rest. An increase in tidal volume is primarily responsible for meeting this need at low to moderate intensities. With high-intensity to near-maximal-intensity exercise, minute ventilation rises steeply to meet the body's need for deeper and/or more frequent breathing. This steep rise in minute ventilation is termed the **ventilatory threshold** and is often used synonymously with the terms **lactate threshold** and **anaerobic threshold**. At this threshold, the body can no longer rely primarily on aerobic metabolism to meet its needs, and anaerobic metabolism becomes the predominant energy system.

Physiological Adaptations to Exercise, Training, and Recovery

Chronic Adaptations to Anaerobic Training

Anaerobic training provokes a variety of chronic adaptations. Within the neuromuscular system, motor cortex adaptations in the brain and neural changes in the spinal cord allow an increased rate of motor unit firing and greater recruitment of fast-twitch muscle fibers, causing higher levels of force generation. These neural adaptations are some of the first to occur.

Increased muscle strength and **hypertrophy** (increased cross-sectional muscle area resulting in larger size) are other main adaptations in anaerobic training. Multiple mechanisms are responsible for hypertrophic adaptations, including increased volume and density of muscle components at the cellular level and increased structural proteins that enlarge muscle fiber diameter.

Anaerobic training causes adaptations in connective tissue, such as increased bone mineral density, increased collagen synthesis, and greater force transmission from tendons, ligaments, and fascia.

Adaptations in the cardiovascular system include increased cardiac output, decreased blood pressure, and decreased resting heart rate; however, these are less substantial than the adaptations that occur with aerobic training.

Chronic Adaptations to Aerobic Training

The main chronic adaptations to aerobic training center around improved cardiovascular function, marked by improved maximal oxygen uptake. Resting heart rate decreases and stroke volume and cardiac output increase, as the heart pumps out a larger volume of blood with each beat. In the respiratory system, tidal volume increases, as the muscles of respiration boost breathing efficiency.

At the muscular level, the capillary density of muscle fibers increases in response to the body's increased demand for oxygen. A greater density of capillaries means greater efficiency in removing carbon dioxide as waste and using oxygen as fuel, since the gases do not have to travel as far to diffuse across cell membranes. Mitochondria increase in size and number, and **myoglobin**, an oxygen transporter, increases as well. In addition, the ability of muscles to use fat for fuel and spare glycogen is improved. These metabolic adaptations lead to increased aerobic capacity and increased aerobic power.

Some muscle hypertrophy also occurs with aerobic training. Adaptations occur primarily in type I muscle fibers due to their high capacity for endurance and resisting fatigue; however, the hypertrophic adaptations are less sizable compared to anaerobic training adaptations.

OVERTRAINING

A physiological stimulus of overload must be applied for training adaptations to occur; however, when the stimulus is too intense or too excessive or recovery is inadequate, **overtraining** can occur, which is a long-term decrease in performance.

There are several types of overtraining, not all of which are automatically negative. **Overreaching**, also called **functional overreaching (FOR)**, is a type of overtraining that nets only temporary performance decreases. It may be planned as part of periodization followed by tapering, where the athlete can quickly recover. This can lead to long-term performance improvements.

Non-functional overreaching (NFOR) refers to the effects of a prolonged, excessive training stimulus paired with inadequate recovery, with impacts that may last for weeks to months. The athlete is likely to exhibit decreases in performance and stamina and increased fatigue.

Overtraining syndrome (OTS) refers to the most prolonged impacts of overtraining, where the athlete can be affected for numerous months. When NFOR is prolonged, such as from too much progressive overload on the body, NFOR can progress into OTS.

SIGNS AND SYMPTOMS OF OVERTRAINING

Overtraining, such as in non-functional overreaching or overtraining syndrome, can cause a variety of physiological and psychological symptoms. The athlete may exhibit stagnation or a decrease in performance, have an increased resting heart rate and blood pressure, become more susceptible to illness, and exhibit disturbances in sleep and mood.

With preventing overtraining, it is important to consider that not all individuals tolerate the same type of overload in the same way. An overload that provokes positive adaptations for one athlete may be an excessive amount of stress for another athlete. In general, with progressive overload, volume and intensity should be gradually increased over time, while avoiding increasing both variables at once. Providing proper recovery time based on the overload stimulus also helps to prevent overtraining by reducing fatigue. Behaviors that support exercise recovery, such as adequate sleep, good nutrition, and stress management, are additional ways to prevent overtraining.

DETRAINING

Detraining is based on the principle of reversibility, where physiological training adaptations will recede or disappear without adequate training stimulus. Detraining may be a temporary necessity, such as pausing or decreasing exercise to recover from illness or injury. Detraining is typically categorized as **short-term** (four weeks or less) or **long-term** (more than four weeks). Longer periods of detraining will have more significant losses in adaptations.

Aerobic endurance is one of the most affected adaptations from detraining, where even short-term detraining can reduce performance. Specifically, VO_2 max decreases due to decreases in cardiac output, stroke volume, and blood volume. With anaerobic adaptations, an athlete may retain their strength performance in short-term detraining; however, long-term detraining can result in decreased strength and muscular atrophy, due to decreased muscle fiber cross-sectional area. Additionally, the number of type IIx fibers increases and the number of type IIa fibers decreases with detraining, reducing the amount of fast-twitch muscle fibers available to recruit.

SLEEP DEPRIVATION AND SLEEP HYGIENE

Sleep deprivation is not getting the amount of sleep the body needs. Adults need 7–9 hours of sleep per night, adolescents need 8–10 hours of sleep per night, and high-performing athletes of any age may require even more sleep. Sleep deprivation may be due to environmental factors (like travel or irregular schedules), behavioral choices (such as stimulant intake or inconsistent bedtimes), or **sleep disorders**, where impaired aspects of sleep consistently affect daily functioning (such as insomnia, sleep apnea, or narcolepsy). There are multiple health and performance implications of sleep deprivation. Cognitive processes may be impaired, lowering motivation, reaction time, and concentration. Physiological impacts include metabolic dysfunction, impaired immunity, and reduced strength, power, and aerobic performance.

Sleep hygiene involves choices or behaviors that promote consistently restful sleep. Sleep measurement tools, such as self-reporting questionnaires, can highlight patterns of sleep disturbances or needs for sleep hygiene strategies. There are two main sleep hygiene strategies: identifying behaviors or environmental factors that promote getting adequate sleep (e.g., limiting caffeine intake or creating a relaxing bedroom environment) and keeping a consistent sleep schedule with a similar wake and sleep time every day.

Recovery from Training

Strategies for recovering from training can be broadly categorized into either refueling depleted muscles or allowing muscles time to recover and repair (including the daily requirement of adequate sleep).

Nutritionally, adequate calories and macronutrients are an essential part of recovery. For example, muscle glycogen cannot be replenished without adequate carbohydrate consumption. Replenishing fluids is also vital for recovery, since dehydration can impair performance, and athletes may require added electrolytes depending on the nature of their activity.

The amount of time needed for muscle recovery and repair is proportional to the amount of muscle used and the intensity. For example, an athlete who has participated in 1-rep maximum attempts may need multiple recovery days, while an athlete who did a submaximal aerobic training bout maybe require less rest. Long-term excessive training (**overtraining**) may warrant multiple days to weeks for recovery. **Tapering**, a planned training volume reduction, may be used as a recovery strategy as well. **Cross-training** is a way to enhance muscle recovery while maintaining physical activity, as it uses different muscle groups than the athlete's given activity. For example, a runner who incorporates swimming for cross-training can maintain their fitness while reducing the amount of repetitive impact and stress on muscles and bones.

Special Considerations of the Differences among Athletes

Biological Age and Training Age

Consideration of **biological age** is necessary in youth to provide accurate evaluations of development and maturity related to fitness and skill. **Biological age** refers to stages of maturation. The most common method of estimating biological age for a strength and conditioning professional are somatic assessments, including height, physique, and limb length. In comparison, **chronological age** refers to age in years or months, which is not always an accurate assessment of a youth's readiness for training. In addition, **training age** refers to the length of time a youth has received supervised resistance training. A youth with a higher training age is likely to have higher skill and competency than a youth who is new to training. Two individuals who are the same chronological age may differ widely in their biological ages and/or training ages and would, therefore, receive different individualized considerations in their program designs.

Resistance Training in Youth

Youth participation in resistance training can net a variety of benefits, including improved muscular strength and endurance, improved power, injury prevention, increased bone mineral density, neural adaptations that improve coordination and skill, reduced sedentary time, and overall improved health and fitness.

Resistance training that is administered safely and effectively has far more benefits than risks for youth; however, there are specific strategies needed to prevent injury. Programs should start conservatively in volume and intensity and allow adequate recovery. Programs should focus on enjoyment, variety, improving skills, and proper technique over competition and specialization, as highly competitive, specialized training can lead to overuse injuries and burnout. One potential injury unique to youth is an **epiphyseal plate fracture**, which is trauma to the growth cartilage at the end of long bones. Using proper instruction, technique, and progression reduces the risk of this injury in youth.

Age-Related Changes in Older Adults

While an **older adult** is typically defined as being over 65, declines in performance begin around age 30. Two musculoskeletal changes with aging are **osteopenia**, or low bone mineral density, and **sarcopenia**, a decrease in muscle mass and strength. Osteopenia can progress to **osteoporosis**, characterized by very low bone density that increases bone fracture risk. Besides reduced muscle mass and strength, decreases in muscle force production and balance are other age-related changes. These changes put older adults at higher risk for falls and loss of functional abilities; however, significant training adaptations can still occur regardless of an individual's age. Older adults benefit from training programs by slowing age-related decline and improving musculoskeletal health.

Training Program Considerations for Older Adults

Before starting a training program, older adults should undergo **prescreening**, which includes getting their medical histories, training histories, and any preexisting medical conditions. This ensures that exercise programs can remain safe and injury-free. Some conditions, such as cardiac conditions, come with higher risk and may require physician clearance before starting any type of exercise. Skill levels and limitations can vary widely across older adults, which often requires careful individualization in their programs. In general, untrained, older adults should start with low-volume, low-intensity exercises using resistance training machines and be allowed adequate recovery (48–72 hours) between sessions. More experienced older adults can progress to exercises that require more postural stability and balance, such as compound exercises using free weights. Training programs should include exercises for flexibility, balance, dynamic stability, and **proprioception** (muscle response to maintain joint stability for the body's sense of position). In addition, the **Valsalva maneuver**, a breath holding technique for core stabilization in weightlifting, should be avoided for older adults as it provokes a rapid blood pressure increase.

Training Program Considerations for Females

Females receive the same benefits from resistance training as males, such as reduced injury and improved health and fitness. However, females will have a lower rate of absolute strength, lower rate of power output, and less muscle hypertrophy due to hormonal differences. Females can build the same quality of muscle and make strength gains at the same rate as males, so females do not need different training programs or exercises than males. The only difference in the training program between the sexes will be the amount of absolute resistance used for exercises.

The **female athlete triad** is a health risk unique to females and occurs due to prolonged training with inadequate calorie intake. As a result, bone mineral density is reduced, increasing the risk of **osteoporosis**. Additionally, menstrual function is impacted, resulting in **amenorrhea**, or loss of the regular monthly menstrual cycle for 3 months or more. The female athlete triad can lead to bone fractures and decreased performance.

One other consideration for females is increased ACL injury risk. Many factors may contribute to this risk, but it can be reduced with balanced, periodized training that incorporates increasing the strength and neuromuscular control of the muscles that act on the knee joint.

Training Status

Training status is the current ability and preparedness of an individual relevant to a training program, which includes injuries, health conditions, and training background. Understanding training status allows the strength and conditioning professional to evaluate appropriate needs and goals to individualize the program. For example, training status is commonly used in resistance training to classify individuals as beginner, intermediate, or advanced. A beginner who is new to resistance training will need detailed and thorough feedback on technique, exercises that require low skill and coordination levels, and a lower training stress (such as lower volume or intensity, longer rest time, and more recovery days per week) so their body can safely adapt. Conversely, an individual with an advanced training status has built the adaptations to train most days of the week and incorporate more technically complex movements at higher intensities and volumes.

Scientific Research and Statistics in the Exercise Sciences

Types of Research Studies

A strength and conditioning professional is likely to encounter various types of research studies used in exercise science, such as studies that assess the effectiveness of training interventions or that provide trends based on data. **Quantitative** research studies use objective, numerical data to investigate comparisons or relationships, such as studying the relationship between consumption of a supplement and strength gains. **Qualitative** research studies use subjective data like observations or interviews to gain more detail on a subject of study, such as why athletes make specific nutritional choices.

Types of studies include **experimental studies** and **descriptive studies**, both of which can be quantitative or qualitative. In experimental studies, a dependent variable is influenced or changed by one or more independent variables. An example is testing a group of athletes before and after a training intervention. The training intervention would be the independent variable, and the amount of muscle or strength gained or lost after the training would be the dependent variable. In descriptive studies, behavior or other variables are observed without external influences. There are many types of descriptive studies. **Longitudinal studies** are where subjects are observed over time for cause-and-effect relationships. **Case-control studies** observe how non-experimental interventions affect outcomes. **Cross-sectional studies** collect data from different groups at one point in time.

Descriptive Statistics

Descriptive statistics provide a summary of the data from a study that creates a description of all individuals who were tested. **Measures of central tendency** show trends in how the data is clustered. The **mean** is the average score based on all individuals' results, and the **median** is the middle score when scores are ranked from lowest to highest. For example, in a program to enhance speed, the mean score of all athletes in a 100-meter dash could be compared before and after the program to evaluate how well the program is working.

Variability refers to how the scores of all individuals tested are distributed. **Standard deviation** is a useful measure of variability and measures how variable scores are relative to the mean. For example, standard deviation could be used to identify athletes whose scores are significantly below the group mean.

Percentile rank is another useful category of descriptive statistics that ranks scores from lowest to highest, allowing identification of where a specific individual's score falls in relation to the scores of others. For example, athletes that score in the 25th percentile have higher scores than only 25% of other athletes and might be identified for additional training or conditioning to boost their percentile rank.

Sources of Information and Evidence-Based Practice

Evidence-based practice means that decisions are made based on the current best scientific evidence. Strength and conditioning professionals need to understand and apply evidence-based practice so that they can make effective, informed, and safe decisions for those they train. Scientific research articles from peer-reviewed journals, academic publications, and official NSCA resources are some of the strongest sources to inform evidence-based practice. These sources present unbiased, objective information and are rigorously reviewed by experts to ensure they are accurate and credible.

Other sources may not be inaccurate but lack scientific rigor. Magazine articles, many websites (such as commercial ones focused on making a profit), many blog posts, and many types of social media content are not the strongest choices to use in evidence-based practice. Information in these sources is not always rooted in science and can be biased toward making sales or gaining followers rather than presenting objective data. There can be exceptions, such as social media posts from a nationally accredited fitness organization (such as the NSCA) that provide a snapshot of new research findings; however, going directly to the scientific research resources that the post is based on would be the ideal choice.

Inferential Statistics and Effect Size

Inferential statistics allow inferences, or general conclusions and predictions, based on data. Inferential statistics are grounded in the assumption that the **sample** (the group that underwent the testing) accurately represents the **population** (the entire larger group to which the sample belongs). If a strength and conditioning professional is evaluating the implementation of a new training technique, they can use existing research with inferential statistics to determine the technique's effectiveness. The strength and conditioning professional should seek studies with a sample that is similar to their own target population, based on factors like sex, age, sport, experience level, and others.

Effect size provides a quantifiable determination of how strong the relationship is between two given variables or between before-and-after testing. General effect size guidelines provide 0.2 as a small effect, 0.6 as a moderate effect, and 1.2 or more as a large effect. A strength and conditioning professional evaluating research on various similar training techniques could look for the effect size and select the training technique with the largest effect size across research.

Test Reliability

Reliability is the degree to which a test produces consistent or repeatable results. For example, a body composition method that gives a measurement with 0.01% difference across multiple measurements for the same athlete would be much more reliable than a measurement that differs within 5%. **Test-retest reliability** is one way to determine reliability of a test and involves giving the same test multiple times to the same athletes. A test with high reliability should result in similar scores every time.

Test reliability can be improved through consistency on both the subject's part and the tester's part. **Intrasubject variability** is the variance within an individual's performance. An athlete may produce a less reliable score due to psychological factors, like low motivation or stress, or physical factors, like fatigue levels. **Interrater reliability** is the degree of consistency in agreement across different testers, and **intrarater reliability** is the degree of consistency within the same individual tester. Testers should be trained in measurement details for competency to boost test administration reliability.

TEST VALIDITY

Validity is a test's ability to accurately measure what it is designed to measure. For example, a VO_2 max test has high validity for assessing aerobic capacity, while estimating VO_2 max with an equation has lower validity because it is not a direct measure. There are four types of validity that warrant further consideration in testing. **Construct validity** is the degree to which a test accurately represents the construct it is designed to measure. If a test lacks construct validity, all other types of validity will be affected. **Face validity** is an informal, subjective element where the test appears to measure what it is supposed to, which can enhance motivation in the test subject to do well on the test. **Content validity** is the degree of expert assessment with which the test has been developed with respect to all relevant abilities. Content validity is especially relevant in a battery of multiple tests to ensure that all important components are covered. **Criterion-referenced validity** refers to test score association with a similar measure for the same ability. For example, if two agility tests have similar validity but one takes longer to set up, the less time-consuming one may be chosen.

Sport Psychology

Psycho-physiological Factors of Performance

REINFORCEMENT AND PUNISHMENT

In motivational theory, a target behavior is called an **operant**. Positive and negative reinforcement are both used to increase the likelihood that the operant will occur. **Positive reinforcement** involves providing something perceived as positive after the operant occurs. For example, a coach who wants to foster a spirit of cooperation among athletes might give a 'teamwork award' to athletes who are consistently displaying cooperative behavior. **Negative reinforcement** involves removing something perceived as negative after the operant occurs. For example, athletes who have demonstrated excellent teamwork might be permitted to skip a grueling training drill.

While reinforcement is used to increase the likelihood of an operant (a given behavior), punishment is used to decrease it. **Positive punishment** involves providing something that decreases occurrence of the operant, such as making any athlete who is late to practice run extra laps. **Negative punishment** involves taking something away as motivation to avoid the given behavior, such as an athlete who gets a time-out and a reduction in playing time for unsportsmanlike behavior.

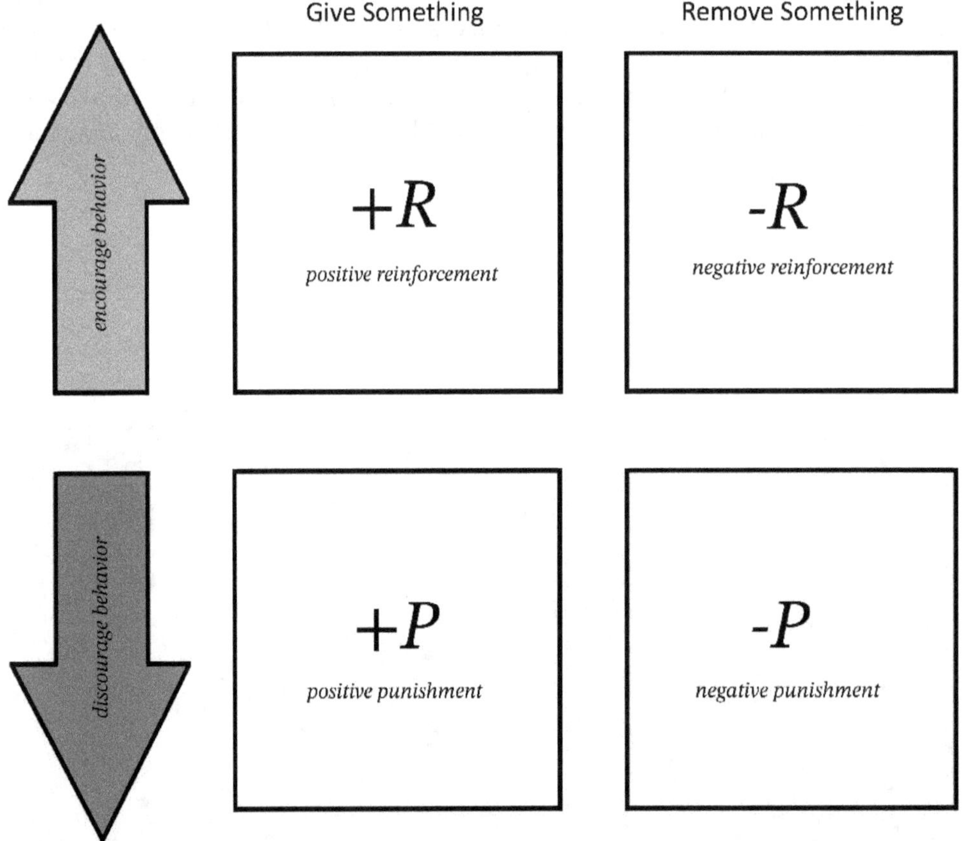

Both reinforcement and punishment may be used to influence an operant, but reinforcement is a more constructive approach as it recognizes desirable behavior, which enhances motivation to perform.

Relaxation Techniques

Relaxation **techniques** are often used to manage arousal, such as decreasing responses associated with anxiety (worry, rapid heart rate, lack of focus, etc.). **Diaphragmatic breathing** increases concentration and focus through directing the breath into expanding the abdominal region through maximal, slow inhalations. This type of breathing enhances the activity of the parasympathetic system, promoting reduced stress. **Progressive muscular relaxation** involves alternating between maximally contracting and relaxing muscles in cycles, proceeding through all main muscle groups. **Autogenic training** involves a focus on relaxing, physical sensations for muscles or body segments. **Systematic desensitization (SD)** uses **counterconditioning**, mental and physical techniques that build coping skills and arousal management for a perceived fearful situation, helping to replace the fear response with a relaxation response instead.

Imagery

Imagery goes beyond visualizing to include all sensory elements to recreate or mentally rehearse an experience. Including details beyond sight, like sounds, smells, or textures creates a more authentic image that transfers into more effective psychological practice. An athlete might use imagery to go through all the steps of an athletic technique from start to finish, helping them mentally experience the actions before executing them. Imagery can be performed from a **first-person perspective** by rehearsing the experience in one's own body or from a **third-person perspective**, as if watching oneself as an observer. Besides helping with mental preparation, imagery can be used to build feelings of confidence and success. Since imagery is within an individual's psychological control, they can manipulate the imagery to create positive outcomes. For example, a weightlifting athlete might use imagery to create all the details of a competition scenario in their mind where they are succeeding at a new maximal lift.

Self-Efficacy

Self-efficacy is an individual's belief in their ability to achieve a specific goal or task. Since self-efficacy is context-specific or task-specific, an individual may have high self-efficacy in one context and lower self-efficacy in another. For example, an athlete may have high self-efficacy for succeeding at training drills in practice but low self-efficacy for performing under pressure. In addition, an individual with higher self-efficacy for a given goal will put forth more persistence and effort toward that goal. Therefore, building self-efficacy is advantageous for performance.

Self-efficacy can be increased through four primary methods. **Mastery experiences**, also known as **performance accomplishments**, are past attainments that reinforce the ability to succeed. **Vicarious experiences** occur through observing and modeling the behavior of others who are successful. **Verbal persuasion** comes in the form of feedback from the self (i.e., self-talk) or others (such as encouragement from a teammate). **Physiological and emotional states** encompass an overall sense of how an individual is feeling, such as high arousal, stressed, confident, etc.

Self-Talk

Self-talk is an individual's inner dialogue. As self-talk often reflects one's beliefs about one's performance, it can influence self-efficacy and have positive or negative impacts. **Negative self-talk** reflects criticism or judgment (e.g., "There's no way I can make this shot"), lowering confidence in abilities. **Positive self-talk** reflects encouraging, productive statements (e.g., "I have trained hard for this moment, and I am ready"). **Instructional self-talk** provides cues or directions (e.g., "Take a deep breath before shooting the ball") and is typically helpful as a mental reminder of a performance focus. An athlete's inner dialogue can be very individual, but in general, negative self-talk is counterproductive to performance. One tactic that can be used to increase negative self-talk awareness is to log or count incidences of negative self-talk over a training cycle or training session.

Counteracting negative self-talk can be done through modifications, such as reframing negative statements into ones that are instructional or positive.

Goal Setting

Goal setting is a process where specific and measurable aspects of a task are defined along with a gradual progression toward achieving that task that is relevant to the individual. Goals must be specific and measurable so that accurate feedback can be provided on progress, reinforcing motivation to persist toward the goal. Goals can be categorized into two broad types based on the amount of control that an athlete has over them. **Outcome goals** are not fully within an individual's control. For example, winning a team championship may not be the best choice for a motivating goal for an individual, since success depends on other people and other factors. **Process goals** are primarily within an individual's control and focus on achievable, consistent actions, such as putting in a set amount of time each week toward extra strength training work. Systematically setting goals can involve combining both outcome and process goals. For example, a swimmer sets the goal to make the varsity team at the end of the season (outcome goal) by attending practice five times a week (process goal).

Arousal and Anxiety

Arousal is an ever-present combination of psychological and physiological activation that exists on a continuum and is neither inherently positive nor negative. The level of ideal arousal for optimal performance is not the same for everyone. **Anxiety** is a subcategory of arousal that has two components—**cognitive anxiety** and **somatic anxiety**. Cognitive anxiety refers to negative emotional states based on perception, like worry, and somatic anxiety refers to physical effects of anxiety, such as sweating or elevated heart rate. Further, anxiety can be conceptualized as a short-term experience (**state anxiety**) or a more enduring personality characteristic that makes one more prone to experience state anxiety (**trait anxiety**). While anxiety may be perceived negatively, it does not necessarily always have negative effects on athletic performance.

Drive Theory

Drive theory is one of multiple theories describing the relationship between arousal and performance. It suggests that arousal has a linear relationship with performance, where the best performance occurs with high levels of arousal; however, this premise is not always true, as high levels of arousal can impair performance. There are two main factors that influence whether higher arousal levels are beneficial for performance—**skill level** and **task complexity**. Athletes with lower skill levels need lower arousal levels to perform at their best, since they are using more cognitive energy to perform effective skills. Complex tasks also benefit from lower arousal levels, as lower levels allow the athlete to focus their attention on the task without high arousal being a distraction. Conversely, simple tasks that do not require constant conscious thought may be enhanced with a higher level of arousal.

Inverted-U Theory and Individual Zones of Optimal Functioning (IZOF) Theory

The **inverted-U theory**, also known as the **Yerkes-Dodson law**, proposes that individuals have an optimal level of arousal and that arousal only enhances performance up to a certain point. Arousal levels that are too low cause performance to suffer, and arousal levels that pass the optimal level can feel debilitating to performance and excessively stressful.

The **individual zones of optimal functioning (IZOF) theory** better accounts for individual differences and factors in responding to arousal compared to the inverted-U theory. The IZOF theory proposes that there is an optimal range of arousal for each individual and that both positive and negative emotions can influence performance—whether for better or for worse. For example, two athletes have elevated levels of arousal because they are excited to play in their first championship game. One athlete's high arousal causes feelings of nervousness and apprehension, which have a negative impact on performance, while the other athlete's high arousal provokes feelings of motivation and focus, which have a positive impact on performance.

Overall, both theories highlight that some extent of arousal enhances performance but that the appropriate level depends on the individual and the context.

Catastrophe Theory and Reversal Theory

Catastrophe theory is another theory describing the relationship between arousal and performance. It is best viewed in contrast to the inverted-U theory, which proposes that there is an optimal level of arousal for performance with a gradual performance decline if exceeding that optimal level. Catastrophe theory poses that there can be a dramatic performance decline with arousal levels that are too high. **Choking** in sports illustrates this dramatic decline, which is described as significantly decreased performance while under pressure. For example, a basketball athlete who is typically an excellent free throw shooter may experience choking and miss all their free throws in a high-pressure game if their arousal is too high. This illustrates catastrophe theory.

Reversal theory states that arousal depends on individual interpretation. Under this theory, two athletes experiencing the same level of arousal may perceive it very differently and have very different performance outcomes. This premise is similar to the individual zones of optimal functioning (IZOF) theory, but reversal theory goes further by explaining that individual perception can be changed and manipulated for more positive impacts on performance. For example, an athlete could be guided into perceiving physiological effects of arousal as motivating and energizing rather than debilitating.

Athlete Mental Health and Wellness

Scope of Practice for Psychological Issues

The **scope of practice** involves what is required professionally and legally from a given role. It is important for strength and conditioning specialists to understand what they can and cannot do from a psychological standpoint in assisting athletes. There are many psychological aspects of sport, and a strength and conditioning specialist can assist with general performance-enhancing activities, such as facilitating techniques for stress management, teaching skills for improved psychological performance, enhancing motivation, and guiding athletes with goal setting.

Psychological aspects that are outside of the scope of practice include providing any type of targeted intervention like therapy or counseling and diagnosing psychological or mental health conditions. It is within the scope of practice (and a professional responsibility), however, to be aware of signs and symptoms of specific issues and have readily available resources to assist affected athletes as needed. For example, a suspected eating disorder or mental health condition like depression should receive a referral to a qualified professional.

Psychological Impacts of Injury

Injuries in sports can have a profound psychological impact on athletes. Athletes facing injuries may experience anxiety, depression, eating disorders, and other mental health issues. Injured athletes may also sense a loss of identity and reduced social support when their injuries limit them from any team participation. Negative or unproductive psychological responses to injuries can complicate the healing process, such as fear of reinjury, lack of motivation, depression, and unrealistic recovery expectations; however, certain psychological reactions can aid in recovery and facilitate a stronger return to sport, such as self-efficacy, self-esteem, and realistic recovery expectations. Overall, it is important for the strength and conditioning professional to consider both an athlete's psychological health along with physical health during injury recovery. Providing support, normalizing emotional struggles, and addressing mental health issues can all be beneficial in reducing negative psychological impacts of injury.

ANXIETY DISORDERS

Anxiety can be a natural response to the stress of performance. In some cases, it can even be beneficial and motivating; however, **anxiety disorders** go beyond temporary worry or fear, and the persistence of these feelings can interfere with regular activities and daily life. While there are several types of anxiety disorders, common signs and symptoms include excessive worry out of proportion to the threat (or when there is no threat), difficulty focusing or sleeping, and physical symptoms such as muscle tension, nausea, sweating, high heart rate, or feeling lightheaded. A rough guideline for distinguishing between a normal anxiety-based response to a stressor and a potential anxiety disorder is to gauge if the anxiety regularly goes beyond sports performance. Anxiety that regularly interferes with daily life may indicate a need for a referral to a mental health professional.

DEPRESSION

Depression is a type of mood disorder, where negative thoughts and feelings persist long-term and interfere with an individual's normal ability to function. Signs and symptoms of depression include negative mood states, low energy, difficulty concentrating, difficulty sleeping or sleeping excessively, changes in weight or appetite, and loss of interest in previously enjoyable activities. Thoughts of death or suicide can also accompany depression, making it vital for strength and conditioning professionals to recognize signs and symptoms of depression to refer athletes out for treatment. While it is not in the scope of a strength and conditioning professional to diagnose or treat depression, one readily available resource is the National Suicide Prevention and Crisis Lifeline, reached by dialing 988. Depressive signs and symptoms can also indicate overtraining, and asking further questions or using screening tools are ways to help distinguish if an athlete may be chronically depressed or simply overstressed and lacking proper training recovery.

EXCESS STRESS

Excess stress can significantly impact performance, both physically and mentally. Physically, stress can manifest with signs and symptoms such as headaches, stomach aches, issues with sleeping, higher resting heart rate, lowered immunity (such as getting sick more often), and changes in appetite (whether eating more or eating less). Muscle tension is another common sign of stress, which may impact motor functions and increase injury risk. Mentally, the signs and symptoms of stress may include feeling irritable or restless, changes in memory (such as forgetfulness), impaired cognition, focus, and learning, and diminished abilities for decision-making and judgment. Over time, excess stress can initiate or worsen mental health disorders such as anxiety and depression. It also puts an individual at higher risk for cardiovascular health conditions. One specific sub-type of stress is **overtraining**, where long-term performance decreases last for weeks or months resulting from excess training and inadequate recovery.

RESTRICTIVE EATING DISORDERS

Individuals with **anorexia nervosa** restrict their eating to such a point where extreme weight loss results. The restriction stems from a fear of weight gain or **body dysmorphia**, where extreme and unrealistic thoughts about one's appearance impact normal function. Ritualistic eating habits may be present, and individuals with anorexia may use binging and purging to further limit their food intake. Starving the body of calories and nutrients can result in symptoms such as osteoporosis, muscle weakness, amenorrhea in females, fatigue, damage to internal organs, and even death if left untreated.

Individuals with **avoidant/restrictive food intake disorder (ARFID)** significantly limit the amounts or types of food they eat, which can progress to having a limited range of preferred foods, dramatic weight loss, and nutritional deficiencies. Unlike anorexia, those with ARFID do not exhibit body dysmorphia or a fear of weight gain.

Eating Disorders Involving Binging

Bulimia nervosa involves repeated episodes (at least once per week for 3 months or more) of binging on large amounts of food and then purging. Purging may occur through vomiting, laxatives, diuretics, exercise, or a combination of these. The binge and purge cycles typically occur in secret and are often accompanied by feelings of a loss of control. Compared to restrictive eating disorders where individuals have low body weights, individuals with bulimia nervosa may be underweight, normal weight, or overweight. Purging methods like vomiting and laxative use can cause gastrointestinal problems, dehydration, and electrolyte imbalance.

The main difference between **binge eating disorder** and bulimia nervosa is that binge eating disorder does not involve purging. Rather, the individual has repeated episodes of binge eating (at least once a week for 3 weeks or more) where they consume significantly more food than normal. Like bulimia, the binge cycles typically occur privately, and the individual may feel out of control, embarrassed, or disgusted with their behavior. Individuals with binge eating disorder tend to be overweight because they are repeatedly consuming calories in excess of the body's needs.

Nutrition

Nutritional Factors Affecting Health

MyPlate and Dietary Reference Intakes

MyPlate (along with the corresponding website MyPlate.gov) is a tool from the USDA that can be used as a resource to estimate nutritional needs. Using the graphic of a place setting, it depicts five food groups (grains, protein, vegetables, fruits, and dairy) along with guidelines on how meals can incorporate all five groups. Athletes can use MyPlate as a starting point to evaluate if they are consuming a diet in line with MyPlate recommendations for their sex, age, physical activity level, and other factors.

Dietary Reference Intakes (DRIs) are helpful in understanding daily values of nutrients based on individual needs. There are four different DRIs. The **Recommended Daily Allowance (RDA)** is the average daily dietary intake meeting the nutrition requirement of nearly all individuals in a given group. The **AI (Adequate Intake)** is used as a daily average when the RDA cannot be established. The **EAR (Estimated Average Requirement)** meets the requirement of half the individuals in a given group. The **UL (Tolerable Upper Intake Level)** is the highest daily nutrient intake not likely to pose risk of adverse health effects.

Protein

Protein is made of amino acids. There are 20 different amino acids required to support cell structure and function. Some amino acids are essential, meaning they must be obtained from food, and some are nonessential because the body can synthesize them. Foods like meat, poultry, fish, eggs, dairy, nuts, and seeds are all sources of protein; however, not all protein-containing foods are of the same quality, since they have different amounts of amino acids and different levels of digestibility. Proteins derived from animal sources and soy are higher quality than plant-based sources because they are more digestible and contain all the essential amino acids.

Protein should make up 10–35% of total calories. The RDA for adults is 0.8 grams of protein per kilogram of body weight. Athletes have higher protein needs to support muscle growth and repair, requiring 1.4 g/kg of body weight to 1.8 g/kg of body weight. Consuming more protein than these amounts is unlikely to cause issues but is not typically necessary. Post-exercise protein consumption is beneficial for athletes because it can enhance muscle protein synthesis. A post-exercise meal should contain a ratio of around 3–4 parts carbohydrates to 1 part protein.

Carbohydrates

There are three main groups of carbohydrates. **Monosaccharides** are single sugars such as glucose and fructose. **Disaccharides** are joined groups of two simple sugars, such as sucrose. **Polysaccharides** are also called complex carbohydrates and are made of many glucose units. Examples include glycogen, starch, and fiber. Sources of carbohydrates include breads, cereals, grains, pasta, vegetables, legumes, and fruits. Health benefits are associated with diets that are high in fiber and other complex carbohydrates and low in refined carbohydrates, such as candy and other highly processed snack foods. Athletes may need to consider the timing of their athletic activities when consuming some types of complex carbohydrates since foods high in fiber can cause gastrointestinal distress when eaten before or during exercise.

Carbohydrates should comprise 45–65% of total calories. Carbohydrate needs for athletes depend on the nature of their sport. Athletes who do aerobic endurance and/or high-intensity intermittent activities may need up to 8–10 grams of carbohydrates per kilogram of body weight daily, and athletes who do more anaerobic activity have lower needs (5–6 g/kg body weight daily).

The Glycemic Index

The **glycemic index (GI)** provides a 1–100 ranking for how high a given food raises blood glucose levels 2 hours after a meal based on digestion and absorption. It can be used to assess several types of carbohydrate-containing foods and help athletes make choices based on their needs. High-GI foods (ranked at 70 or more) are digested and absorbed more quickly. Pure glucose has a GI of 100. Lower-GI foods, ranked at 55 or less, have slower digestion and absorption and tend to be higher in complex carbohydrates. These foods include grains and vegetables.

For athletes, the GI can be a guide in selecting foods based on the immediacy of energy needs from blood glucose. For example, an aerobic endurance athlete doing a very long training session or competition would benefit from higher-GI foods to raise blood glucose rapidly and provide quick energy. Lower-GI foods would not provide the needed blood glucose boost as quickly and would be better choices to eat around non-exercising times.

Fat

There are several types of fats (also known as lipids), and some types of fats are essential for body processes like cell structure and function, hormone regulation, vitamin storage, and energy storage. **Saturated fats** can be made by the body and are not a dietary requirement. **Trans fats** are another type of fat that are not a dietary requirement. They are typically found in processed foods as chemically changed plant oils. The ingredients label will typically indicate them as "partially hydrogenated oil." Consuming foods with high levels of saturated fats and trans fats can have long-term health implications, such as increased cholesterol and weight gain. Fats like **monounsaturated fat, polyunsaturated fat,** and **omega-3 and omega-6 fatty acids** are more desirable choices and can be found in a variety of foods, such as fatty fish, nuts, seeds, and vegetable oils. Fats should comprise 20–35% of total calories. Dietary recommendations for calories from fat include limiting saturated fat and trans fat to 10% of total calories or less.

Dietary Iron

Iron is an essential mineral for the body and is particularly important in athletic performance because it carries oxygen and assists in energy production. Individuals who do not consume enough iron are at risk for performance impacts since low iron means less oxygen to the working muscles. **Iron deficiency** is decreased iron in the body relative to needs. The RDA for males is 7–11 mg, and the RDA for females is 7–27 mg. If iron deficiency persists, **iron deficiency anemia** can result, where oxygen delivery is impaired due to fewer red blood cells. Athletes deficient in iron may have symptoms that affect their performance, such as fatigue, shortness of breath, reduced aerobic capacity, and poor concentration. Females typically require more iron than males, as females store less iron in their bodies and lose blood during the menstrual cycle if they are of menstruating age. Iron can be found in whole grains, leafy greens, and protein-rich foods such as meat, poultry, eggs, nuts, beans, and seeds. **Heme iron** is absorbed better by the body and is found in animal meats. **Non-heme iron** is found in non-meat foods and is absorbed less effectively.

Calcium

Calcium is an essential mineral for the body that is critical in maintaining bone health and enabling muscle contraction. Consuming enough calcium is particularly important for young athletes who are still growing so that they can develop strong bones. For mature adults, adequate calcium is vital for maintaining bone density levels. The RDA for calcium is 1,300 mg for teenagers, 1,000 mg for males 19–70 years old and females 19–50 years old, and 1,200 mg for males over 70 and females over 50. Long-term failure to consume enough calcium can compromise bone health. **Osteopenia** is an early stage of losing bone density, which can progress to **osteoporosis**, where bones become porous and brittle, increasing the risk of bone fractures. Good sources of calcium include dairy products, such as milk, yogurt, and cheese, and non-dairy products that have been fortified, such as plant-based milk or fortified juice. Soy products and leafy greens are also calcium-rich sources.

Maintaining Fluid Balance

Maintaining hydration is particularly important in athletic performance because fluids and electrolytes can be lost in sweat. **Dehydration** is the process of losing water from body functions, and **hypohydration** is the resulting decreased amount of water in the body. These may cause performance impairments, like the perception of exercise as being more difficult, increased heart rate, and a reduction in most if not all aspects of fitness, including endurance and strength. Additionally, dehydration and hypohydration increase susceptibility to heat stress, such as heat stroke, due to increased core temperature.

Attaining the Adequate Intake (AI) of water can help to maintain fluid balance. The AI of water for males is 3.7 liters per day, and the AI for females is 2.7 liters per day. This does not have to be solely attained through water; any fluids from other beverages and foods go toward the AI. Some populations may be at higher risk for dehydration or need more fluids than the AI, such as children, older adults, individuals new to training, individuals who sweat profusely, and individuals training in high-temperature or humid environments.

Fluid Intake Guidelines

Losing as little as 2% of body weight through water loss can impair performance, highlighting the importance of preventing dehydration in athletes. Hydration status and sweat rate can be assessed through pre-workout and post-workout weighing to determine fluid needs.

In some situations, plain water is not enough to restore body fluids. Individuals who sweat profusely or do prolonged, intense exercise can benefit from also replacing electrolytes, such as sodium and potassium, which can be done through sports drinks or food. Otherwise, **hyponatremia**, a dangerously low dilution of sodium in the blood, can result. Symptoms of hyponatremia include muscle cramping, nausea, vomiting, and even risk of coma and death.

Specific hydration needs depend on factors like age, sweat rate, and environment, but the following are general guidelines. Prior to activity, athletes should prehydrate so that they do not begin their activity under-hydrated. During activity, athletes should follow an individualized plan for the amount of water they regularly consume. The athletes' potential need for electrolytes should also be considered. After activity, athletes can replenish fluids and electrolytes through normal eating and drinking but may need added fluid with electrolytes if they have lost significant weight through sweat.

Nutrition to Maximize Performance

Metabolism and Calorie Requirements

Individuals wishing to change their body composition (whether gaining lean muscle or losing body fat) should start with estimating their daily caloric needs. There are three components that contribute to daily caloric needs. The first one is **basal metabolic rate (BMR)**, which is the energy the body needs to sustain normal functions like breathing and brain activity. BMR is often used synonymously with **resting metabolic rate (RMR)**, which is slightly higher and reflects the energy needed in a resting state. BMR and RMR are the largest contributors to daily caloric needs at 65–70% or more. **Thermic effect of food** is a second contributor to daily calorie needs and reflects the energy required by actions like eating and digesting. **Physical activity** is the third contributor to daily caloric needs and the most easily manipulated. If comparing two individuals of the same sex, age, weight, and height, the more active person will require more daily calories. Prediction equations like the **Harris-Benedict equation** or **Cunningham equation** can be used to estimate RMR and then factor in physical activity level to provide an approximation of an individual's daily caloric needs.

Nutritional Strategies for Weight Gain

Athletes may wish to gain weight for various reasons, from building lean muscle to improve performance to regaining weight lost after a prolonged illness or injury. Adding around 500 extra calories per day is a general strategy to promote weight gain while mitigating gaining excess body fat. The surplus calories should come from nutrient-rich foods with a balance of all three macronutrients—carbohydrates, proteins, and fats. Dietary protein is particularly beneficial for increasing lean muscle. Consuming 1.5–2.0 grams of protein per kilogram of body weight daily will support weight gain goals. Drastically increasing calorie consumption can be challenging, so athletes can benefit from an initial 100–200 extra calories a day and increasing over time. The extra calories can be spread throughout daily eating in the form of larger meal portions and/or more frequent snacks. Athletes may also benefit from guidance from a qualified nutrition professional to support their weight gain goals.

Nutritional Strategies for Weight Loss

In a simple sense, weight loss is achieved through having a regular caloric deficit, or consuming fewer calories than what the body would normally need; however, there are multiple factors and individual variations that influence weight loss. Athletes can achieve caloric deficits in many ways. There is no single best diet that works for every athlete. Choosing to replace high-calorie foods with lower-calorie, nutrient-dense foods, reducing calories from added sugar and fat, and reducing alcohol consumption are all possible strategies to elicit a caloric deficit. The most significant nutritional predictors of successful long-term weight loss are total caloric intake and adherence to the diet over a long time.

The average caloric deficit is often given as 500 calories per day, which is equal to losing about a pound a week, yet a smaller daily caloric deficit can still be effective over time. Diets and methods that result in weight loss greater than 1–2 pounds a week should be avoided because they may be unsustainable or the weight lost may be from body water or lean muscle. To maximize weight loss from body fat and preserve lean muscle, athletes with weight loss goals should consume 1.8–2.7 grams of protein per kilogram of body weight.

Fad Diets

A **fad diet** is one that promotes quick, easy results to change body composition or weight while lacking scientific evidence for its effectiveness. Fad diets are often highly restrictive, eliminating one or more food groups, or require other drastic dietary changes. Some examples of common fad diets include juice fasting, detoxification diets, and the Atkins diet. In juice fasting, an individual consumes only beverages such as juices or smoothies. However, this diet can leave people feeling hungry due to the lack of protein and fiber, both of which are satiating. Detoxification, or "detox" diets, take many forms but have the underlying premise of "cleansing" the body through strict elimination of many types of foods and/or fasting. These are not long-term solutions for weight management, and someone is likely to regain weight once they stray from the diet. The Atkins diet significantly restricts carbohydrates, emphasizes high protein, and promotes the company's own processed products, such as shakes or bars. Since the body needs carbohydrates for energy, a low-carbohydrate diet can leave an individual feeling weak and sluggish. The most effective approach to weight management is one that an individual can sustain, which is not typically the case for fad diets.

Pre-Competition Nutrition

The main goals of pre-competition nutrition are to maintain fluid and energy levels for performance and minimize gastrointestinal distress. General guidelines include eating small quantities closer to the start of competition, consuming foods that are moderate in protein and low in fat and fiber, and consuming familiar foods and drinks rather than trying new things. Consuming foods high in carbohydrates can be particularly beneficial for aerobic endurance athletes and may benefit other types of athletes. The composition of meals and snacks can vary depending on the athlete and the nature of their sport.

There are, however, general guidelines for timing pre-competition nutrition to achieve optimal performance. Prehydrating in the hours leading up to competition is an important strategy. Some athletes may need to eat 4 hours before competition to minimize gastrointestinal distress, with the meal comprising 1–4 grams of carbohydrates per kilogram of body weight and 0.15–0.25 grams of protein per kilogram of body weight. Meals consumed 2 hours before competition should be smaller and comprise 1 gram of carbohydrates per kilogram of body weight. For nutritional intake 1 hour before competition, quick-digesting carbohydrates, like sports drinks or gels, are good choices for optimal performance. These should provide 0.5 grams of carbohydrates per kilogram of body weight.

Carbohydrate Loading

Carbohydrate loading involves consuming high amounts of carbohydrates starting a few days before a competition or event. The premise is that the extra carbohydrates allow the body to store more glycogen, reducing fatigue and enhancing performance. Carbohydrate loading often starts 3 days before the targeted event. During a carbohydrate loading phase, an athlete consumes around 8–10 grams of carbohydrates per kilogram of body weight daily. For some athletes, daily caloric intake may need to increase to accommodate the extra amount of carbohydrates.

Athletes doing aerobic endurance activities can benefit most from carbohydrate loading since the long duration of their activities can deplete glycogen otherwise; however, athletes doing other activities may also benefit from carbohydrate loading. While various foods can be used to implement carbohydrate loading, it may be best for athletes to avoid foods high in fiber, especially on the night before competition and on the day of competition. Foods high in fiber take longer to digest and can cause gastrointestinal distress. Carbohydrates that are digested quickly, such as white bread, bagels, rice, and pasta, are typically a better choice to use in carbohydrate loading.

Nutrition During Competition

Many types of activities do not warrant additional nutrition or hydration (other than plain water); however, hydration is important during events in hot and humid conditions or during events where an athlete is sweating profusely. Athletes in these situations can benefit from consuming sports drinks containing 6–8% carbohydrates. This replenishes electrolytes and prevents water loss. Water loss of 2% or more can negatively affect performance.

Nutrition during competition is particularly important when events are longer than 45 minutes (such as aerobic endurance activities), when there are prolonged bouts of high-intensity exercise, and when an athlete has multiple events in a day. In these cases, athletes may benefit from consuming carbohydrates through a sports drink containing 6–8% carbohydrates and/or through food that is easily digested, such as gels or bars. Not all types of carbohydrates are transported and utilized in the exact same way by the body, so one recommendation is to consume a combination of carbohydrates to maximize what the body can use and absorb.

Post-Competition Nutrition

The main goals of post-competition nutrition are to repair muscle tissue and replenish glycogen, fluids, and electrolytes. Methods to accomplish these goals can vary widely depending on individual needs and the nature of the activity, making it challenging to provide exact amounts of macronutrients for every situation; however, general guidelines for athletes to accomplish these goals include drinking water, eating normally, and considering adding sodium and/or a sports drink if they have lost a substantial amount of fluid. Athletes in glycogen-depleting activities like aerobic endurance events should consume carbohydrates and protein within the first two hours after exercise. Athletes in other types of sports, like intermittent high-intensity activities and strength and power activities should also consume protein after their sports, as this aids muscle protein synthesis for tissue repair. If they are going to participate in their sports again within 24 hours, these types of athletes will also benefit from replenishing muscle glycogen through higher carbohydrate consumption.

Nutritional Needs Based on Performance Goal

Nutritional needs vary based on performance goals such as endurance, strength, and hypertrophy. For endurance athletes, the focus is on carbohydrates, electrolytes, and fluids to optimize fueling during long-duration activities. Carbohydrates play a crucial role in providing sustained energy. Endurance athletes are recommended to consume 8–10 grams of carbohydrates per kilogram of body weight daily. Sports drinks with multiple types of carbohydrates can be used to replenish fluids and electrolytes. Protein intake for endurance athletes is advised at 1.0–1.6 grams per kilogram of body weight daily to support muscle repair and recovery.

Strength athletes have higher protein requirements compared to endurance athletes, with the recommended range at 1.4–1.7 grams per kilogram of body weight daily. Post-exercise protein consumption is particularly emphasized to enhance muscle protein synthesis. Supplementing with carbohydrates should be considered before and during competition to maintain muscle force and reduce muscle fatigue.

For hypertrophy, it is recommended that an athlete eats protein more frequently to support protein synthesis and build muscle mass. Athletes focused on hypertrophy should consume 20–30 grams of protein every 3–4 hours. After a training session, supporting muscle repair and protein synthesis can be accomplished by consuming 40 grams of protein and 30–100 grams of high-glycemic carbohydrates.

Measures of Weight and Body Composition

Body composition refers to the proportion of fat-free mass and fat mass within the body. Fat-free mass includes muscles, bones, and body water, while fat mass includes subcutaneous fat under the skin and visceral fat surrounding organs. Body composition can be measured through methods such as skinfolds or a DEXA scan.

Body mass index (BMI) and waist circumference are two common ways to estimate body size, though they do not provide information on body composition. **Body mass index (BMI)** is a person's weight in kilograms divided by the square of their height in meters. A normal BMI is usually considered to be between 18.5 and 24.9, overweight is between 25 and 29.9, and obese is between 30 and 34.9. Higher BMIs are associated with higher risk of disease. BMI may be less useful for athletes with high amounts of muscle mass, as it may place them in the overweight or obese categories based on weight alone. **Waist circumference** is measured at the level of the navel. Higher measurements indicate greater amounts of visceral fat, which carries more health risks. Females with a waist circumference over 35 inches and males with a waist circumference over 40 inches are at higher risk for disease.

The Impact of Alcohol and Drugs

Alcohol

Alcohol does not have any benefit in enhancing performance, though athletes might choose to use it to promote feelings of relaxation and calmness before their activity or after their activity to socialize or celebrate. Alcohol is a depressant, so signs and symptoms of alcohol use are often related to the inhibition or slowing down of body processes. These may include sleepiness, impairments in memory and attention, and reduced coordination and balance. Some individuals may show increased aggression.

Binge drinking is defined as consuming about 4 drinks or more within 2 hours for females and consuming about 5 drinks or more within 2 hours for males. More significant impairments result when consuming higher levels of alcohol, like in binge drinking. These may include signs of alcohol poisoning, such as vomiting, confusion, mood changes, and slowed breathing. Misusing alcohol in excessive amounts can cause loss of consciousness, coma, and death from suppressed vital body functions.

Short-Term and Long-Term Effects of Alcohol Use

Short-term effects of alcohol use will depend on an individual's blood alcohol content (BAC), which results from the amount of alcohol they have consumed. Consuming alcohol of any amount can hinder performance. At low BACs, implications for performance include slower reaction time, dehydration, impaired judgement, and impaired motor function. At higher BACs, an individual may have severely impaired balance and gait. Alcohol consumption can be deadly if a person's BAC rises high enough (about 0.4%). Short-term consumption of alcohol after exercise can cause dehydration, delaying recovery. Excessive alcohol consumption can cause a hangover, leaving an athlete feeling fatigued and unable to perform optimally.

There are many long-term, chronic effects of alcohol use with implications for performance. Excess calories from alcohol can crowd out nutrient-dense foods, negatively impacting body composition and causing nutritional deficiencies. Consuming excessive alcohol over a long period can also lead to liver inflammation and disease, weakening of the heart muscles, impaired immune system function, and increased risk for multiple types of cancer.

Stimulant Drugs

Stimulant drugs increase activity of the central nervous system and include caffeine, ephedrine-containing products, prescription stimulants, cocaine, amphetamine, and methamphetamine; however, not all stimulants are the same in terms of potency, effects, and legal status in sports. For example, caffeine at normal consumption levels is permitted in sports and less likely to be problematic, while illicit drugs are not permitted and pose a higher risk of misuse and abuse.

In an athletic context, stimulants can enhance performance by making an athlete feel more alert and focused while reducing feelings of fatigue. Signs and symptoms of stimulant use include rapid heart rate or heart palpitations, feelings of anxiety or panic attacks, trouble sleeping, headaches, and increased risk of heat stroke.

Misusing stimulants over a long period can result in addiction and tolerance, where the user craves the drug and needs increasing amounts to get the same effect or to function normally. Long-term use can also impact the cardiovascular system, leading to hypertension, heart attack, and stroke.

Supplements and Performance-Enhancing Substances

Ergogenic Aids

Ergogenic aids are anything used to improve performance. Athletes who select supplements or other performance-enhancing substances to use as ergogenic aids should be aware of making informed choices. Not all ergogenic substances are legal or permitted for performance. Some, like illicit drugs, are illegal on a national level, while others are substances banned by athletic organizations. Athletes should be aware of the rules governing their particular sports and countries so that they are not barred from competing.

Athletes should also be aware that most, if not all, supplements and performance-enhancing substances have health risks, even if the risks are small. The claims for a supplement may not always be true. Objective scientific research is helpful in guiding decisions regarding whether the benefits outweigh any potential risks.

Proper periodization in training, including recovery, and good nutrition are the first steps in supporting performance over supplementation. Athletes should have solid foundations in these before considering how supplements or other substances will fit into maximizing their athletic potential.

Supplements

The Dietary Supplement Health and Education Act (DSHEA) specifically states what can be classified as a **supplement**. This definition includes:

- The item must be intended to be ingested as a liquid, powder, or pill/caplet/capsule
- It is not marketed as food
- It clearly marked as a dietary supplement
- It is intended to increase the regular intake of a particular vitamin or mineral
- It is a concentrated version of the vitamin or mineral, a metabolized version, a part of a vitamin or mineral, an extract of a vitamin or mineral, or a mixture of these components
- It is a nontobacco product with at least one of the following: a mineral, a vitamin, some plant product, or an amino acid compound

Supplements are used to augment a diet in which some component is missing or lacking.

Supplement Considerations

First and foremost, a person should discuss his or her nutritional and dietary needs with a **licensed dietitian** or **physician** before beginning any course of supplementation. Tests can be performed to check for deficiencies, and patient/physician can engage in a dialogue about what is needed and how to go about obtaining that. Results can vary, and are dependent on the person's physical and mental state and the quality of the supplement.

A person should research the brand and company that is producing the supplement. Because supplements are not regulated in the same manner as drugs and the FDA does not check the accuracy of the claims made, it is essential that a person uses a trusted brand with safe products.

Amino Acids

The body requires 20 different amino acids, 8 of which are essential amino acids that must come from food. The remaining 12 amino acids can be made by the body. Out of the essential amino acids, three are **branched-chain amino acids (BCAAs)**—leucine, isoleucine, and valine. These are key amino acids for muscle protein synthesis and a common supplementation choice for athletes. Research shows that BCAAs may benefit muscle recovery and do not appear to have adverse effects; however, since BCAAs are found in protein-containing foods, athletes should first focus on consuming adequate calories and protein before considering BCAA supplementation.

Beta-alanine is another amino acid commonly used in supplementation. It is often included in pre-workout formulas. Its main premise is to increase type II muscle fiber function through influencing carnosine synthesis, thus improving anaerobic performance. Research has found a positive relationship between beta-alanine supplementation and anaerobic threshold but not maximal strength or aerobic power, so it is most suitable for high-intensity, intermittent activity. Other amino acids have less evidence for performance enhancement. For example, **arginine** is purported to cause **vasodilation** (widening of blood vessels) through increasing nitric oxide levels; however, this does not appear to lead to improvements in athletic performance.

Creatine

Creatine is one of the most widely used and well-researched ergogenic aids. Its effectiveness in enhancing performance has been shown in a large number of studies. Creatine is synthesized in the body and can also be obtained from animal sources like meat and fish. Creatine phosphate (CP) is vital in forming ATP, and when CP stores decrease, performance declines from fatigue. Supplementing with creatine helps maintain stored amounts of creatine in the muscle to sustain high intensities during exercise.

Creatine supplementation has been shown by research to improve strength, recovery, power, and muscle mass, though not all individuals respond the same to creatine supplementation. It has little to no significant side effects besides mild gastrointestinal disturbances in some athletes. It is important to note that an effective regimen of creatine supplementation involves loading the muscles with extra creatine stores and then maintaining the stores. This can be done through consuming 0.3 grams of creatine per kilogram of body weight for 5–7 days followed by a maintenance dose of 2 grams daily for as long as desired. Alternatively, the athlete could start at the maintenance dose and reach full saturation within around 30 days. Consuming carbohydrates and protein with creatine can increase the amount of creatine the muscles absorb. Stopping the daily dose does not result in an immediate decrease in muscle creatine levels. Rather, a decrease occurs after about 4 weeks of stopping use.

Stimulants

There are a variety of stimulant drugs that vary in potency, effects, and legality. Some (like caffeine) are permitted within limited amounts by sporting organizations and carry a lower risk of negative effects. Other stimulant drugs are legal in some contexts but prohibited in sport, and others are illegal.

Ephedrine is a stimulant drug that raises metabolism, promotes fat loss, and improves aerobic endurance. Ephedrine is often an ingredient in cold and sinus medicines because it also dilates the breathing passages, reducing congestion. It can, however, have negative effects like vomiting and nausea and is banned in most sport contexts.

Athletes might choose illegal stimulant drugs, such as cocaine or amphetamines, as ergogenic aids to feel less fatigued and more focused and alert. These are not only against the law but are banned by sports organizations. Negative health implications for performance can include heatstroke, impaired judgment, distorted reality, irregular heartbeats, and even death. Additionally, illegal stimulant drugs can be highly addictive due to influencing the brain's neurotransmitters and can cause intense withdrawal effects when their use is stopped.

Caffeine

Caffeine is a commonly used and well-researched ergogenic aid. It functions as a central nervous system stimulant to reduce fatigue and maintain performance levels in addition to increasing alertness and mood. For aerobic athletes, it can improve endurance and time to exhaustion. For anaerobic athletes, it can increase muscular strength and anaerobic power. For aerobic athletes, it may enhance power production, but this seems to depend on the training status of the athlete.

Athletes should be aware that caffeine can be addictive and has potential side effects. Consuming caffeine regularly and then stopping can cause unpleasant withdrawal symptoms like headache, decreased mood, and fatigue. Side effects include trouble sleeping, anxiety, irregular heartbeat, and others.

Additionally, athletes choosing to use caffeine should be aware of guidelines for dosing and timing. The most performance-enhancing effects result from consuming 3–9 milligrams of caffeine per kilogram of body weight about an hour before exercise or during exercise of longer durations. Consuming more than 9 milligrams per kilogram of body weight does not have additional effects and can make side effects more likely. Capsules or tablets with caffeine are more powerful than drinks or foods containing caffeine, including gels.

Blood Doping

Blood doping involves increasing the mass of red blood cells through artificial means. This is accomplished through infusing the body with additional red blood cells or taking the drug **erythropoietin** to stimulate more red blood cells to form. The premise of using blood doping as an ergogenic aid is that more red blood cells mean more oxygen transported to muscles, reducing time to fatigue, and improving VO_2 max. Aerobic endurance athletes are the ones most likely to benefit from the effects of blood doping.

Blood doping is banned by the World Anti-Doping Agency (WADA), so any athlete found using blood doping methods can be barred from competition. Additionally, blood doping poses significant health risks. Higher levels of red blood cells thicken the blood, increasing the risk of cardiopulmonary events like embolism, stroke, and heart attack. While blood doping can indeed improve performance, the risks of being prohibited from competing and incurring health issues far outweigh any benefits.

Anabolic Steroids

Anabolic steroids are synthetic variants of the sex hormone testosterone. While testosterone is found in both males and females, the much higher levels in males contribute to them having more muscle mass and greater strength levels. Therefore, the premise behind using anabolic steroids is to further increase muscle mass and strength beyond the body's normal abilities. Besides strength and power athletes, steroids may be used by individuals who desire to improve their appearance through hypertrophy, such as bodybuilders. There are several types of anabolic steroids, which are either administered orally or through injection.

Anabolic steroids are banned by most major sport organizations, including the World Anti-Doping Agency (WADA). Anabolic steroids pose significant psychological and physical health risks. Users of steroids are likely to be more aggressive and irritable and experience mood swings. Physically, anabolic steroids affect many different body systems. In the cardiovascular system, increased blood pressure, altered blood lipid levels, and decreased heart function may result from anabolic steroid use. Injecting steroids can lead to infections and the transmission of bloodborne diseases. Effects on the reproductive system include testicular atrophy in males and masculinization characteristics in females. Overall, self-administering steroids for performance enhancement reasons is a high-risk choice that is best avoided.

Diuretics

Diuretics are substances that promote increased urine production in the body. Some hormones have naturally diuretic effects as part of normal body processes; however, an athlete may choose to use diuretics as an ergogenic aid. Diuretics are most often used in a sports context for rapid weight loss, such as in sports where making a weight class is important, like wrestling or weightlifting. Another common use for diuretics is to increase urine output to mask the presence of banned substances. Diuretics are banned by most major sports organizations, including the World Anti-Doping Agency (WADA). There are, however, legitimate medical uses for diuretics. Individuals with high blood pressure may be prescribed diuretics to lower the volume of fluid going through the cardiovascular system.

In a non-medical ergogenic aid context, diuretics carry multiple risks. Because they reduce the body's water content, the frequent use of diuretics increases the risk for dehydration and heat illness. Losing weight rapidly through diuretics can result in a loss of muscle tissue, increased fatigue and headaches, and decreased blood pressure and blood volume. In worst-case scenarios, diuretics can significantly alter the body's electrolyte balance to the point of causing kidney failure, irregular heartbeats, and even death.

Program Design

Needs Analysis

EVALUATION OF THE SPORT

MOVEMENT ANALYSIS

Performing a **movement analysis** for a given sport gives detailed insight into aspects like preparatory and dynamic movement patterns, the main muscles and joints involved in those patterns, types of muscular contraction (concentric, eccentric, isometric), needed ranges of motion and planes of motion, and movement velocity. Movement analysis can be done using visual observation, photos, videos, and more specialized, high-tech methods like computerized motion analysis.

Using volleyball as an example, a movement analysis would reveal the following aspects:

- The typical preparatory position is a general athletic 'ready' position with the feet about hip-width and the knees bent.
- Main dynamic patterns include multi-directional running, jumping, diving, and upper body movements to hit the ball.
- Heavily recruited muscles include all major lower body and upper body muscles with both concentric and eccentric contractions, along with the spinal and abdominal muscles assisting isometrically for stability.
- Volleyball particularly requires full ranges of motion in shoulder flexion and extension for serving and spiking the ball.
- All planes of motion are used in volleyball, with sagittal plane movements being the most common.
- Volleyball also requires rapid acceleration, rapid deceleration, and high levels of force production.

PHYSIOLOGICAL ANALYSIS

A **physiological analysis** for a sport is used to indicate whether strength, power, hypertrophy, or muscular endurance (or a combination) is the main priority. Determining this establishes an understanding of the main energy systems used in the sport—whether the phosphagen system, the glycolytic system, the oxidative system, or a combination of these.

Volleyball, for example, requires strength, power, and endurance, fueled by a combination of all three energy systems. Volleyball includes high-power, rapid movements, such as spiking, blocking, and serving. These are fueled primarily by the phosphagen system. A large component of normal gameplay is volleying the ball back and forth over the net to score points, working at higher intensities interspersed with brief recovery. Working for longer periods while still using anaerobic energy systems is primarily fueled by anaerobic glycolysis. Although reacting to the ball in volleyball tends to use brief, explosive movements, volleyball requires some measures of muscular endurance since games are typically played in multiple sets and the entire gameplay can last 60–90 minutes or more. Longer-duration exercises like volleyball are primarily fueled by the oxidative system.

Injury Analysis

Injury analysis uses knowledge of the sport and information from the movement analysis to determine common sites and reasons for injuries. Using volleyball again as an example, the frequent running, jumping, landing, and rapid changes of direction mean that ankle and knee injuries are common. As volleyball players consistently use their arms for force production in serving or spiking the ball, injuries at the shoulder and rotator cuff are also common. The wrists and fingers are also vulnerable to injuries like sprains or dislocations from coming into contact with the ball or other players.

While not all injuries can be prevented in sports, this information is particularly helpful in reducing the incidence of overuse injuries from repetitive movements and reinforcing correct form and technique. For example, the information from this injury analysis could be used to consistently reinforce proper running, jumping, and spiking patterns in practice through various techniques, as well as creating proper stabilization by supporting muscles to reduce injury risk.

Evaluation of the Athlete

Training Status

Training status is the level of current conditioning or preparedness of an athlete before beginning a program. Aspects of training status include current or previous injuries; previous background of training in the sport; history of all prior training; frequency, intensity, duration, and type of training; and the knowledge and skill of exercise technique.

Athletes can be broadly classified into one of three categories based on their training status, though this information should be used as a generalization and not an objective measurement. A **beginner** is someone who is untrained or began training less than 2 months ago, trains at low intensities and low frequencies, and has minimal experience with proper technique. **Intermediate** indicates that the athlete has been currently training a few times a week at medium intensities for 2–6 months and has some basic knowledge and familiarity with proper technique. An **advanced** athlete has been training for over a year on most days of the week, doing demanding workouts and demonstrating a high level of skill in proper technique. Overall, evaluating training status must be individualized to the athlete. For example, an advanced athlete returning from a serious injury is less prepared for the full demands of the sport than an uninjured athlete.

Physical Testing and Evaluation

Physical testing and evaluation provide an objective way to evaluate where an athlete's qualities may be strong and where they may be lacking relative to the needs of the sport. There are physical tests for all health-related components of fitness (cardiovascular endurance, muscular endurance, muscular strength, flexibility, body composition) and tests for all skill-related components of fitness (agility, balance, coordination, power, speed, reaction time). Most, if not all, sport contexts use multiple components of fitness, so typically a sequence of multiple tests would be performed for a comprehensive scope of the athlete's abilities.

Movement analysis should be used to guide testing choices for an athlete. For example, a movement analysis for volleyball would indicate that testing for components like muscular strength, flexibility, agility, coordination, power, and reaction time are all useful based on the needs of the sport. To select one specific example from these, let us say that a volleyball athlete is tested for lower body power using the vertical jump test. The athlete's results can be compared to normative data from research or compared with data from other team members to determine if their lower body power is adequate or if it needs improvement.

PRIMARY RESISTANCE TRAINING GOAL

The primary resistance training goal may seem similar to the physiological analysis in evaluating an athlete's needs since it assesses whether strength, power, hypertrophy, or muscular endurance is the priority; however, the primary resistance training goal takes not only the physiological analysis into account but includes the movement analysis as well as individual results from testing and priorities for the season. The priority for the season is a vital aspect because it will direct the nature of the training to help the athlete peak in performance and avoid injury. For example, volleyball athletes in the offseason might have general muscular endurance goals as a priority to attain or maintain a base of fitness before entering more specific, intense training. During the preseason and in-season, priorities will shift to focusing more on strength and power, as these are more directly relevant to the demands that will be encountered in recurring volleyball games.

Training Methods and Modes

TRAINING TO MAXIMIZE PERFORMANCE AND MINIMIZE INJURY

RESISTANCE TRAINING

Information from the needs analysis, particularly the movement patterns of the sport and injury analysis, should be used to guide the selection of resistance training modes and movements. One broad objective where resistance training is commonly used is to enhance stability. For example, sports with repetitive overhead arm movements that require large amounts of force generation, such as baseball, softball, tennis, and volleyball, will all benefit from having some type of consistent scapular stabilization movements as part of resistance training. Otherwise, lack of stability in joints that support the shoulder can lead to overuse injuries and chronic conditions like shoulder impingement. Another example of enhancing stability is incorporating core stability regularly into resistance training. Core stability is important in every sport because a stable core enhances the body's ability to transmit and withstand force. It also helps prevent low back injury and improves balance.

PLYOMETRIC TRAINING

Plyometric training is beneficial across a variety of sports to increase muscle force production and power. Plyometric exercises can be useful for injury prevention when done with proper progressive overload since the body's adaptations will include strengthened muscles and connective tissues such as tendons and ligaments. Plyometrics can mimic or exceed the demands of the sport so that body structures are resilient enough to withstand the often-unpredictable stresses encountered in the sport directly. For example, in sports that require jumping and landing, such as basketball and volleyball, using plyometrics can reinforce using proper alignment at joints, like keeping the knees over the toes. In sports that require single-leg movements, like soccer or running, unilateral plyometrics like single-leg hops and bounds can be used to improve stability and single-leg balance, reducing the risk of knee injuries. In sports that require trunk rotation and explosive upper body movements, like tennis, baseball, and softball, plyometric movements like medicine ball throws and catches can increase the velocity generated by the upper body by coordinating force generation from the core muscles to the limbs.

FLEXIBILITY TRAINING

Most sports require a combination of flexibility and strength to execute movements optimally and to maximize force development and production. For example, Olympic weightlifting requires powerful triple extension to execute the lifts successfully, which is not possible unless the hips, knees, and ankles have adequate mobility and flexibility to fully extend. Some sports, like gymnastics and figure skating, require ranges of motion beyond normal joint flexibility to enhance the execution and artistry of movements for scoring.

Using the movement analysis and injury analysis are particularly important in determining flexibility training methods for a given sport. For example, hamstring strains are common in sports that require sprinting, so focusing consistently on hamstring flexibility and mobility may be preventative. As another example, repetitive high-velocity throws, such as in sports like baseball and softball, place stress on the shoulder and elbow joints. Maintaining flexibility throughout the muscles that act on the shoulder can improve throwing mechanics and distribute the stress over a greater area, reducing risk of injury.

Combining Training Modes to Maximize Power Production

Maximizing power production requires a combination of specific resistance training and plyometric training. Resistance training for power is typically done at 75–90% of 1-RM for 1–5 repetitions. The heavier weight and fewer repetitions recruit fast-twitch muscles over slow-twitch muscles, enhancing muscle force production needed for power. Olympic lifts and their variations are particularly good for goals of maximizing power because they involve higher movement velocities than traditional weight training movements, enhancing muscle ability to rapidly accelerate and produce force.

Doing only resistance training is not optimal for power production, as the movement velocity at near-maximal weights is not very high. Therefore, incorporating plyometric training will enhance the body's ability to transmit forces quickly against lighter resistance. For example, lower body resistance training can be paired with upper body plyometrics on a given training day and then vice versa on the next training day. **Complex training** is another way of incorporating plyometrics that involves doing high-intensity resistance training followed by plyometrics, such as a bench press followed by an explosive medicine ball pass.

Combining Training Modes to Maximize Aerobic Endurance

According to the principle of specificity, the most effective modes for aerobic endurance are ones that primarily rely on the oxidative system, use aerobic metabolism, and are done at lower intensities and for longer durations. One example is **long, slow distance (LSD)** training, where a moderate-intensity workload is maintained at about 60–70% of VO_2 max. LSD is important for building training volume without high stress that would necessitate longer recovery time; however, high-intensity training should also be combined with LSD to improve aerobic performance, such as **tempo training** and **high-intensity interval training (HIIT)**. These are done at higher intensities than LSD—from the lactate threshold to near-maximal levels—and improve both anaerobic and aerobic metabolism. They are also time-efficient.

Cross-training and resistance training also are valuable to combine toward an aerobic endurance goal for injury prevention, muscle balance, and muscular endurance. **Cross-training** is the use of alternate aerobic modes from the primary mode, such as a runner doing cycling and swimming. Resistance training for an endurance goal is typically done at 12+ repetitions, at low intensities (<67% of 1-RM), and over multiple sets with short (30–60 second) rest times.

Combining Training Modes to Maximize Muscle Hypertrophy

The foundation of **muscle hypertrophy**, or building increased lean muscle mass, is resistance training done at moderate intensities (67–85% of 1-RM) for 6–12 repetitions at high volumes (3–6 sets) with short rest periods (30–90 seconds). Training modes for hypertrophy often involve a combination of compound, multi-joint exercises and single-joint exercises. Modes that use multiple large muscle groups increase muscle hypertrophy through the recruitment of numerous motor units to produce force. Single-joint exercises isolate smaller muscle groups to maximize their force production and muscle hypertrophy. Common modes to develop muscle hypertrophy include free weights and machines; however, anaerobic training can be combined with resistance training to maximize muscle hypertrophy. More specifically, plyometrics, speed training, and agility training use type II muscle fibers, which have a higher potential for hypertrophy.

Select Exercises

Structural Exercises and Power Exercises

Structural exercises are ones that load the spine, requiring postural stabilization muscles to be active throughout the movement. Postural stabilization muscles include muscles of the trunk and spine, such as the transverse abdominus, multifidus, external and internal obliques, rectus abdominus, erector spinae, and quadratus lumborum. These muscles work together to keep the body in alignment and control its motion. Examples of structural exercises include deadlifts, squats, bent-over rows, and standing overhead presses. Structural exercises are relevant to all types of sports and activities since postural stabilization accompanies real-life dynamic movement. Movements that do not load the spine, such as using weight machines for a seated overhead press or a leg press, have less direct application to sports-specific movements.

Some structural exercises can be performed explosively or at high speeds. These are considered **power exercises**. The Olympic lifts (clean and jerk, snatch) and their variations (hang cleans, hang snatches, and push jerks) are all examples of power exercises. If a sport does not prioritize explosive movements, power exercises may not be applicable. For example, power exercises would be less relevant to aerobic endurance sports like long-distance running and cycling.

Core Exercises and Assistance Exercises

A **core exercise**, also known as a **multi-joint exercise**, is one that uses two or more joints and one or more large muscle groups. Such exercises can be performed with only bodyweight, such as a pull-up, dip, or lunge, or with external resistance, such as a barbell deadlift or a dumbbell overhead press. An **assistance exercise**, also known as a **single-joint exercise**, uses only one joint and, therefore, typically a smaller muscle area. For example, a biceps curl involves movement only at the elbow joint, and a leg curl (also known as hamstring curl) involves movement only at the knee joint.

In dynamic movement in sports, the body does not typically use single joints in isolation, so assistance exercises have less direct relevance for performance. Therefore, core exercises are the preferred priority in an athlete's plan regardless of the sport; however, assistance exercises have particular use in preventing and rehabilitating injuries. These exercises can focus on weak or injury-prone areas, isolating them to build strength and stability. For example, a runner might do side-lying leg raises to strengthen the hip abductors, improving knee alignment and reducing overuse injury risk.

Closed Kinetic Chain and Open Kinetic Chain Movements

In a **closed kinetic chain movement**, the involved extremities have their distal ends fixed to a stationary surface, such as the ground. Squats, deadlifts, push-ups, and standing calf raises are all examples. In an **open kinetic chain movement**, the distal ends of the involved extremities can move freely. This freedom of movement may involve contact with external resistance, such as with a leg extension machine or doing a lateral raise holding dumbbells.

Closed kinetic chain movements are typically more relevant to functional movements and sport-related movements. They also tend to be multi-joint, promoting stability during dynamic movements. For example, jumping and running require force generation against the ground, so a squat (closed kinetic chain movement) would have more direct application than a leg extension (open kinetic chain movement). This is not to say that open kinetic chain movements are not useful. They can be part of a well-rounded training program and used to isolate single joints to promote injury prevention and rehabilitation. For example, an athlete who lacks strength in the posterior chain may benefit from the open kinetic chain movement of a lying leg (hamstring) curl.

Exercise Selection Based on Application and Movement

Some examples of common movements in sports include jumping and landing, running, throwing-related movements, and rotation. Analyzing the most common movement patterns of a sport should provide insight into which exercises will be the most similar and therefore the most relevant. For effective jumping and landing, an athlete must generate force to leave the ground and land with a stable base. Power exercises (such as the Olympic lifts) and squats would be prime choices in emphasizing lower body force production. For unilateral lower body movements like running or jumping from one leg, unilateral exercises such as lunges, step-ups, and abduction/adduction directly transfer into enhancing single-leg stability. Considering bilateral versus unilateral movement is an important step in selecting throwing-related exercises. Many sports, such as basketball or volleyball, involve both, so using both bilateral and unilateral movements (such as chest press or shoulder press) would be relevant. Sports that require repetitive unilateral throwing or striking, such as baseball and tennis, benefit from exercises that use shoulder extension and/or enhance shoulder stability, such as a pullover or overhead press. Many sports are multidirectional and benefit from rotational exercises. For example, rotational throws or chops are relevant for football, baseball, and golf.

Example: Exercise Selection for Volleyball

A needs analysis for volleyball reveals that this sport requires vertical jumping, multidirectional running, and multidirectional upper body movements, including frequent shoulder flexion and extension. Exercise selection for vertical jumping should prioritize multi-joint movements that require high levels of force production. Any type of loaded squat and deadlift would be directly relevant, as would Olympic lifts like the hang power clean. Multidirectional running engages all lower body muscles and involves unilateral movement, such as during changes of direction. Enhancing stability at the knees and ankles would benefit running technique and assist in injury prevention, with exercise examples including lunges, step-ups, and assistance exercises such as hip abductions and calf raises. Movement at the upper body in volleyball primarily involves horizontal and vertical pushing, with relevant exercises including push-ups, chest press, and shoulder press. Power exercises like the push press or push jerk would also be beneficial to enhance upper body force production. Assistance exercises to strengthen the rotator cuff muscles would also be fitting to enhance shoulder stability during explosive movement and prevent injury. Lastly, upper and lower body plyometric movements (jumps, passes) would benefit explosive power needed in volleyball.

Exercise Selection to Promote Muscle Balance

Muscle groups work in agonist and antagonist pairs to execute movement. **Muscle balance** is an appropriate ratio between the agonist and antagonist relative to each other. These ratios vary depending on the agonist/antagonist pair and are not necessarily equal. For example, the knee extensors and knee flexors are commonly reported to have a ratio of 3:2. Ratios could be measured with isokinetic testing, but lack of muscle balance may also be noticed in 1-RMs for major lifts. For instance, an athlete whose 1-RM deadlift and back squat are similar may be lacking knee extensor strength. The strength and conditioning professional may select exercises (such as single-joint, isolation exercises) that promote muscle balance for a weaker muscle group.

Another application of muscle balance is in an injury prevention capacity. Activities with repetitive movements, such as running and throwing, can cause the agonist muscles to shorten from having to repeatedly generate force, potentially leading to overuse injuries. Ensuring that the antagonist muscles are consistently included in the exercise selection can help promote muscle balance and reduce injury risk.

Exercise Selection to Promote Recovery

Recovery is a necessary part of training for a sport and should be intentionally incorporated into program design. While complete rest is sometimes necessary, recovery can be "active" through movements that minimize stress on the body and are restorative in nature. These movements or exercises are typically done at lighter loads and lower intensities and/or enhance full ranges of motion. For example, a recovery or deload week done after a cycle of heavy resistance training might include intensities at no more than 55% of 1-RM for weighted movements along with a greater focus on bodyweight exercises. Recovery from cardiovascular training could involve lower-intensity activity and/or **cross-training** (using alternate forms of aerobic exercise to minimize stress on often-used muscle groups). Recovery through movement can also involve modes that enhance mobility and flexibility. For example, self-myofascial release, stretching, and modes like yoga can all be used to improve blood flow to muscles by moving through varied ranges of motion without imposing intense stimuli upon them.

Principles of Exercise Order

Exercise Order Based on Training Goals

The main goal when deciding exercise order, regardless of the training goal, is for the athlete to have the ability to elicit their best effort, force capabilities, and technique to complete the exercises successfully. High-intensity and/or technically demanding exercises are typically performed most successfully as the first exercises, as the athlete is not yet fatigued from additional exercises. For example, if an individual's training session is all lower body exercises, including back squats, leg extensions, leg curls, dumbbell lunges, and seated calf raises, the back squat is done first because it is the heaviest and most technically demanding due to the nature of barbells as free weights requiring full-body stabilization.

Some goals warrant deviating from this general principle. An individual training for hypertrophy may use a **pre-exhaustion** technique to enhance muscle growth. In pre-exhaustion, a single-joint exercise is used to fatigue muscles before they are used in a multi-joint lift. For example, leg extensions may be done prior to a back squat. Another example is the goal of building sports-specific muscular endurance. Since athletes may need to perform in a fatigued state, higher-intensity movements may be placed later in the workout to simulate this, such as doing weighted squat jumps after other multi-joint lower body exercises.

Power, Core, and Assistance Exercises

Power exercises require not only high levels of force production and skill but also place high cognitive demands, requiring concentration on technique. Performing these when fatigued can lead to technique errors and higher injury risk. If power exercises are included in an athlete's program, they should be done first (after the warm-up). If there are multiple power exercises in a program, the most technically complex ones should be done first. For example, if an athlete is doing both a snatch and a push press, the snatch should be prioritized as the more physically and cognitively demanding exercise.

In general, core exercises should precede assistance exercises. Otherwise, an athlete will not perform as well on the core exercises due to smaller muscle groups being fatigued in the assistance exercises.

ALTERNATING EXERCISES

Examples of alternating between upper body and lower body exercises could involve doing a shoulder press, then weighted lunges, then push-ups, and then squats. Examples of alternating exercises between agonist and antagonist muscles could involve doing a set of chest presses followed by a set of rows. This is also an example of alternating exercises by their function (push/pull).

These methods can make the exercise session more time-efficient since one muscle group can rest while a different muscle group is working. Moving through exercises for multiple muscle groups with minimal rest (called **circuit training**) can be particularly beneficial for muscle endurance goals. Alternating exercises is also a useful strategy for novice individuals who may only be training a few times a week. By alternating exercises, a full-body workout can be achieved in less time and at a lower intensity. Without implementing alternating techniques, a full-body workout can require an extensive amount of time for rest periods and/or more frequent training days each week.

SUPERSETS AND COMPOUND SETS

A **superset** involves working opposing muscle groups (agonist/antagonist) back-to-back with minimal rest. For example, an athlete might perform a bent-over row and then go directly into a dumbbell chest press. Other common superset pairings are the hamstrings and quadriceps or the biceps and triceps. A **compound set** involves doing two exercises in a row for the same muscle group. For example, an athlete might do a dumbbell chest press and then a flat dumbbell fly. Both exercises use the pectorals as the agonist. Compound sets are most often used in muscle hypertrophy goals. Most major muscle groups involve multiple muscles or muscle segments, commonly known as muscle heads. For example, the quadriceps are four muscles, and the triceps has three heads. Therefore, doing multiple exercises for the same muscle group targets different muscles, heads, angles, and ranges of motion, leading to more optimal muscle development. Both supersets and compound sets are more advanced resistance training techniques, since the minimal rest increases the intensity.

VARYING EXERCISE MODES WITHIN AN INDIVIDUAL PROGRAM

Most sports require, or benefit from, multiple exercise modes to enhance performance. For example, although the foundation of a long-distance runner's training should be running, their performance will also benefit from including resistance training, high-intensity interval training, and other modes. Consider volleyball as another example. This sport involves explosive power and force production with jumping and striking, speed and agility on the court, and a good foundation of strength and endurance. To adequately develop all of these, priorities need to vary throughout the program's cycles, with corresponding modes varying as well.

In general, demanding and intense modes (such as plyometric, agility, and sprint training) should not occur on consecutive days of the week, and there should be 48–72 hours of recovery time between them. Here, recovery does not necessarily mean total rest but time spent at lower intensities. Explosive training and strength training are also modes with potential conflict since fatigue from heavy resistance training could impair explosive performance if the same muscle groups are used. There should be 48–72 hours of recovery between strength training and explosive training sessions.

Varying Energy Systems Training Within an Individual Program

Many sports require athletes to use multiple energy systems to meet the demands of the activity. Sports like basketball, soccer, volleyball, and hockey can involve brief, intense bursts of near-maximal activity along with lower-intensity, longer-duration movement. All energy systems are active simultaneously, but their dominance changes over a range of time rather than at precise points; however, the body's adaptations differ depending on the energy pathway, so varying modes should be done intentionally and systematically with this in mind for the priorities of the athlete, sport, and season. For example, some sports start off their seasons of training by building an aerobic base, where the oxidative system is the priority and used most in cardiovascular training. As athletes move closer to the competitive parts of their seasons, energy system priorities may need to shift to focusing on short bursts of explosive power and speed, using primarily the anaerobic energy system. In this situation, the oxidative system is still important, but it is not the main priority, so aerobic modes may be interspersed as recovery from more intense, anaerobic training days.

Determine and Assign Exercise Intensities

Using RPE to Assign Intensity

Rating of perceived exertion (RPE) scales provide a subjective way for athletes to self-rate their intensity. The most common scale is a 1–10 scale, where 1 is being at rest with no intensity and 10 is a maximal effort. In general, on the 1–10 RPE scale, 3–4 corresponds with a light to moderate intensity, and 5–7 corresponds with a vigorous intensity. In cardiovascular activities, an RPE range can be used to guide athletes to the desired intensity for their training goals. For example, an athlete doing steady-state training may be instructed to not exceed a 4 on the RPE scale.

For resistance training activities, the RPE scale can be used in comparison to a 1-RM, where 1 is very light with little to no effort, and 10 is a maximal effort, or 1-RM, where the athlete could not do more repetitions or more weight. In the middle, a 5–6 on this scale corresponds with the athlete being able to do 4–6 more repetitions. RPE can be used in resistance training to regulate effort without overtraining. For example, an athlete instructed to work at an 8 on the RPE scale should have 2 more repetitions in reserve in a given set.

Using Heart Rate Methods to Assign Intensity

There are two main methods for assessing heart rate, though these rely on estimates of maximal heart rate. **Percentage of maximal heart rate** is 220 minus the athlete's age (termed the **estimated maximum heart rate**) and multiplied by the desired intensity range. In general, moderate-intensity activity is 64–76% of the estimated maximum heart rate, and vigorous activity is 77–93% of the estimated maximum heart rate.

The other method to assess heart rate is the **Karvonen method**. It also begins with subtracting the athlete's age from 220; however, it differs from the previous method in that the resting heart rate is also subtracted. This number is their estimated **heart rate reserve**, or HRR. The HRR is then multiplied by the desired intensity ranges, and the resting heart rate is added back in to each value. In the Karvonen method, 40–60% of HRR is moderate-intensity activity, and 60–90% of HRR is vigorous activity.

Heart rate methods can be used to ensure the athlete is working hard enough toward the desired goal and not overworking. For example, in HIIT training, an athlete may be instructed to work at 80–90% of their HRR, with recovery heart rate below 60% of HRR.

Assigning a Training Load Based on 1-RM or Goal Repetitions

Assigning a training load based on 1-RM requires that the athlete has previously performed an accurate 1-RM. Doing a true maximal lift is only appropriate for experienced intermediate to advanced athletes; however, an estimated 1-RM can be used to prescribe loads when an athlete's activity or training status does not warrant going through the significant physical stress of a 1-RM test. For example, aerobic endurance athletes like long distance runners would not need to go through 1-RM testing for their sport. A 1-RM could instead be estimated based on multiple repetitions. Once a 1-RM is known or estimated, data tables or prediction equations can be used to provide corresponding repetitions based on the percent of the 1-RM, which can be used to assign load. For example, 10 repetitions correspond with 75% of 1-RM.

Not all exercises lend themselves to 1-RM testing. Core exercises (such as squat, deadlift, bench press, and strict press) can handle 1-RM loads, but exercise movements that are single-joint **assistance exercises** would not use a 1-RM. Assistance exercises could be prescribed load through **goal repetitions** instead, with repetition range based on the training goal, such as 12–20 repetitions for a muscular endurance goal.

Testing the 1-RM

A 1-RM test is only appropriate for experienced weightlifters and requires proper safety procedures, such as having one or more spotters and/or having space to safely drop the weight. It is ideal if the athlete has a good estimate of their 1-RM so that testing can be completed in 3–5 testing sets, reducing excessive fatigue that could interfere with testing.

The athlete should do some type of light, dynamic, movement-specific warm-up for 3–5 minutes and then warm up by doing the selected lift at 5–10 repetitions at an easy, light resistance (about 50% of the 1-RM). After a 1-minute rest period, the next warm-up load should be around 70% of the 1-RM with 3–5 repetitions performed. After a 2-minute rest period, the weight is increased to about 85–90% of 1-RM with 2–3 repetitions performed. The athlete rests 2–4 minutes, then the load is increased further with a single repetition performed. The cycle of 2–4-minute rest and gradual loading with a single repetition is repeated until the 1-RM is found. Failure at a given load will require decreasing the weight to an amount between the failed lift and the last successful lift.

Assigning Loads in Resistance Training

Muscular Strength, Muscular Hypertrophy, and Muscular Endurance

After determining if the main priority for the training session or training cycle is muscular strength, hypertrophy, or endurance, an assignment of load (using 1-RM) and corresponding goal repetitions can be provided. For a strength goal, the load should be greater than or equal to 85% of 1-RM with goal repetitions less than or equal to 6. For a muscular hypertrophy goal, the load should be between 67–85% of the 1-RM with goal repetitions between 6 and 12. For a muscular endurance goal, the load should be less than or equal to 67% of the 1-RM with goal repetitions greater than or equal to 12. Using the correct load and rep range toward a specific goal will best create adaptations in the body toward that goal. For example, an athlete training for strength who is lifting far less than 85% of his 1-RM and can do 12 or more repetitions at the weight is not working at a stimulus that will promote optimal strength adaptations. The weight would need to be increased so that the muscles receive appropriate overload for a strength goal.

Power

Percentages for power in resistance training are a unique consideration that are different from strength, hypertrophy, or muscular endurance. This is because maximal power occurs when lifting light to moderate weights at intermediate velocities. Loads that are too heavy will not allow the force generation and velocity needed to develop power. For example, a 1-RM requires a maximal strength effort but cannot be moved quickly.

Sports requiring power typically also require a foundation of strength to initiate high-velocity movements. Therefore, while assigning loads for power training may be one part of an athlete's program, training for strength should not be neglected. For example, a football athlete may have assigned power loads for the hang clean but assigned strength loads for the back squat, deadlift, and bench press.

Determine and Assign Training Volumes

Volume-Load

Volume-load equals the number of sets multiplied by the number of repetitions in the set and the load (weight) lifted in each repetition. For example, if an athlete performs 3 sets of 5 back squats at 200 lb (91 kg), the volume-load is 3,000 lb (1,361 kg).

There are numerous ways to manipulate volume-load, whether for an increase or decrease. For this back squat example, let us say an increase is desired. First, the load lifted could be increased while maintaining constant sets and reps. For instance, the athlete could squat 220 lb (100 kg) for 3 sets of 5 reps, for a total volume-load of 3,300 lb (1,467 kg.). This is a 10% increase, which effectively increases volume-load without increasing injury risk. Another option is to increase the reps while keeping the sets and weight constant. If the athlete performs 3 sets of 6 reps at 200 lb (91 kg), the volume-load is 3,600 lb (1,633 kg). A third option is to increase the sets while keeping the reps and weight constant. In this case, adding a fourth set would result in a volume-load of 4,000 lb (1,814 kg).

Repetition-Volume

Repetition-volume equals the total number of repetitions performed during a given workout. If an athlete does multiple sets, then the sets multiplied by the repetitions results in the total repetition-volume. Let us say that an athlete does 4 sets of 4 depth jumps in a plyometric training session. Their repetition-volume is 16. Since repetition-volume does not take load into account, it is an appropriate way to measure volume for movements that are not resistance-based, such as plyometric and agility drills or speed intervals.

Repetition-volume can be manipulated in a few different ways. First, either the repetitions or the sets could be changed, whether increased or decreased. Let us say in the depth jump example that a decrease in repetition-volume is desired for a recovery week. Doing either 3 sets of 4 jumps or 4 sets of 3 jumps results in a repetition-volume of 12. Another manipulation would be to increase or decrease the frequency of sessions per week. If the athlete is currently doing plyometric training three times a week, a decrease down to two times a week would reduce the repetition-volume over the entire week.

Varying Training Volume to Benefit Performance

Athletes training for strength and power may have relatively low volume compared to an athlete training for hypertrophy, but the near-maximal loads or intensities in training sessions can be even more of a physiologically stressful stimulus. Varying training volume within a given week is one approach. This can be done through having 1–2 'heavy days' with a counterbalance of 'medium' or 'light' days. For example, an Olympic lifting athlete might have one 'heavy day' each on the snatch and the clean and jerk with near-maximal lifting, and the remainder of their weekly training days have core and assistance exercises that are not done at near-maximal loads. The counterbalance of training volume can also be used for modes like plyometric training or high-intensity interval training. If these are done at near-maximal efforts or high intensities, any resistance training on that day should be at lighter loads, though training volume can be preserved by doing additional sets and reps. This approach of varying training volume within the week helps preserve the high quality of high load training days, where the athlete can maintain optimal technique without being overly fatigued or experiencing overtraining.

Quantifying Training Volume for Cardiovascular Training

One way to apply training volume to cardiovascular training is **metabolic equivalents (METs)**. Existing MET values from research state that one MET equals the body's oxygen cost at rest, 3–6 METs is moderate intensity, and 6+ METs is vigorous intensity. These numbers are broad ranges. MET values for specific activities can be calculated from VO_2 max testing or estimated through existing MET data. Training volume can be measured in MET minutes per week or MET hours per week. If an athlete is training at 4 METs for 5 hours a week, their MET volume for that week is 20 hours.

Training volume for cardiovascular activity can also be evaluated in distance. For example, in sports like running, rowing, cycling, or swimming, training volume can be quantified as the sum of an athlete's total distance per week (whether in meters, miles, yards, etc.). This total can be evaluated in progressing the training program to ensure that volume increases are gradual to avoid overtraining. In general, distances should not increase by more than 10% from week to week. For example, an athlete who is currently running 60 miles a week can increase to 66 miles the next week.

Training Volume for Muscular Endurance, Muscular Hypertrophy, and Muscular Strength

Training volume for muscular endurance prioritizes fatigue-resistant muscles through performing higher repetitions with lighter loads. The training volume for muscular endurance is 2–3 sets of 12 or more repetitions. Training volume for hypertrophy uses moderate loads and the highest volume compared to muscular endurance or muscular strength. The high volume maximizes muscle fiber recruitment and metabolic stress to stimulate growth in muscle mass. The training volume for hypertrophy is 3–6 sets of 6–12 repetitions. In addition, maximizing muscle growth involves performing three or more exercises per muscle group. High volumes with multiple exercises can make for a long workout, so it is common that those training for hypertrophy perform a **split routine** where different muscle groups are trained across different days rather than a full-body workout in one day. Training volume for strength uses the heaviest loads at near-maximal intensities but lower training volume than hypertrophy. The training volume for strength is 2–6 sets of 6 or fewer repetitions.

Training Volume for Power

Training volume for muscular power is 1–2 repetitions over 3–5 sets for a single-effort event (such as Olympic weightlifting or track and field events). For a multiple-effort event, like team sports requiring power, such as volleyball or football, the training volume is 3–5 repetitions over 3–5 sets.

The volume for power is typically lower than the volume required for other goals (muscular endurance, muscular hypertrophy, and muscular strength). While the loads may be near-maximal for a given lift (such as 80–90% for the 1–2 repetitions), power movements are not ones that are done at maximal strength intensities, as overly heavy loads would prevent the velocity needed for power development. For example, an athlete's maximal clean may only be about 50–60% of their deadlift. Overall, the high velocities with maximal force production required for power training dictates that the volume remains relatively low. If the athlete becomes fatigued from too many repetitions or sets, the quality of power exercises can suffer, leading to a breakdown in technique and potential injury.

Determine and Assign Work: Rest Periods, Recovery and Unloading, and Training

Rest Periods in Resistance Training

Rest periods in resistance training depend on the specific training goal and what adaptations are desirable to elicit. In muscular endurance training, the overall goal is to increase the muscle's ability to sustain continuous submaximal contractions over longer durations. Therefore, rest periods for this goal are the shortest—typically 30 seconds or less between sets or exercises. The goal in muscular hypertrophy training is to increase muscle size. Rest periods of 30–90 seconds maintain stimuli that promote muscle size, such as growth hormone, while still allowing sufficient recovery for proper technique. Training for muscular strength focuses on increasing near-maximal to maximal amounts of force generation by the muscles. Longer rest periods of 2–5 minutes are recommended to allow full recovery of the neuromuscular system at these high intensities. For muscular power, the goal is to improve the speed at which force can be generated. Power movements in resistance training also warrant longer rest periods of 2–5 minutes to ensure neuromuscular recovery between sets or reps.

Work-to-Rest Ratios in Aerobic and Anaerobic Interval Training

Work-to-rest ratios are vital in aerobic and anaerobic training because they determine the effectiveness of the workout by accounting for the intensity of the work. Rest periods can mean total rest or active recovery, such as jogging at low intensities. In aerobic interval training, generally recommended ratios of work to rest range from 1:1 to 1:3. This allows for recovery while still maintaining an elevated heart rate that improves the body's use of oxygen. For anaerobic training, maximal to near-maximal intensities require the longest rest periods. Intervals done for 5–10 seconds at peak intensity warrant work-to-rest ratios in the range of 1:12 to 1:20. For example, a 10-second, all-out sprint may require over a minute and a half of rest. Intervals done at high intensities, such as for 15–30 seconds, may use a work-to-rest ratio of 1:3 to 1:5. Overall, rest intervals that are too short decrease the quality of effort and increase risk of overtraining, but rest periods that are too long may reduce the desired challenge to the aerobic or anaerobic system.

Training Frequency Across Seasons

Training frequency is the number of training sessions in a given time period, typically one week. Adjusting frequency throughout a season is important for optimizing peak performance and preventing overtraining. The following are general guidelines across four sport seasons (off-season, preseason, in-season, and postseason), though the needs of the individual and/or sport may dictate different training frequencies.

In the off-season, training frequencies can be their highest, at 4–6 sessions per week. This is the time to build a foundation through base training with longer durations and lower intensities, which need less recovery. This makes a higher training frequency possible. In the preseason, intensity typically increases, warranting more recovery time and lower frequency, such as 3–4 times per week. During the in-season, the focus shifts to sport-specific skills and competition, and a frequency of 1–3 times per week accommodates adequate recovery to maintain peak performance. In the postseason, a typical training frequency can range from 0–3 times per week. An athlete may need total rest to rehabilitate injuries; otherwise, the focus is on maintaining fitness through lower duration, intensity, and frequency.

Influences on Resistance Training Frequency

Training Status and Fitness

The training status and fitness level of an individual are two of the biggest factors that determine training frequency. Individuals who are new to resistance training or have a lower fitness level (such as significant time off from previous training) should start with a frequency of 2–3 times per week. Training days should be non-consecutive with at least one recovery day (but not more than three) between sessions. This lower frequency allows for adequate recovery and adaptation. As fitness improves, individuals with an intermediate level of experience and skill with training can train 3–4 times per week. To avoid training the same muscle group on two consecutive days and to maximize volume, a **split routine** may be used, such as training lower body on Monday and Thursday and upper body on Tuesday and Friday. This allows for greater volume and intensity, promoting further improvements. Advanced individuals who are highly trained with extensive experience can handle high frequencies because they have a higher recovery capacity. They may train up to 4–7 times per week or even have multiple workouts per day.

Other Factors

Apart from individual fitness and training status, several other factors can influence the frequency of resistance training. Different training goals require different training frequencies. For example, someone with a hypertrophy goal should train each muscle group multiple times per week to attain enough training volume for growing muscle mass. In contrast, a novice individual training for muscular endurance can receive benefits with only two sessions per week. In addition, a training goal like strength requires near-maximal effort, so additional recovery time may necessitate offsetting frequency.

The sport season also influences training frequency. For example, during the in-season, priority may be given to sport skill development and recovery from competition instead of frequent resistance training. Additional training, such as plyometric training and anaerobic interval training, also influences training frequency, as high-intensity workouts of this nature may require lower resistance training frequency for recovery.

Lastly, individual aspects like injury history, recovery ability, occupation, time constraints, and stress may require short-term or long-term adjustments in frequency. For example, a student athlete experiencing psychological stress during finals week may need a temporarily lower frequency than usual to avoid putting additional stress on the body's systems.

Influences on Aerobic or Anaerobic Training Frequency

A main consideration for training frequency in aerobic or anaerobic training is the balance between frequency, volume, and intensity. High-volume and high-intensity workouts typically require long recovery periods, reducing training frequency. Conversely, if a high training frequency is desired, then volume and intensity should be moderated to avoid overtraining.

Like the frequency of resistance training, the frequency of aerobic and anaerobic training also depends on the goal, athlete status, training season, and individual factors. With goals as an example, an athlete training in multiple modes (such as for a triathlon) will need high frequencies and even multiple workouts per day to devote training time to each mode. With athlete status, beginners often benefit at a lower frequency (compared to more advanced athletes) to allow recovery and adaptation. Regarding training season, frequency may decrease in the in-season from the preseason to offset the higher intensity and needed recovery of competitions or races. Time is one example of an individual factor that can influence frequency. A person's schedule may not accommodate long training sessions on most days of the week, so they may choose to lower the weekly frequency but have days with higher volume, such as long, slow distance (LSD) training.

Determine and Assign Exercise Progression

Mode Progression

A key factor in determining the appropriate mode or modes for an athlete is how directly they transfer into improving performance at the chosen activity. For example, a long-distance runner should have running as the foundation of their training program, with resistance training and flexibility training as supplements to promote muscle balance and prevent injury. In general, logical progression of modes goes from more basic or foundational to more complex or skilled. Steady-state, low-intensity modes are a starting point for the foundation of sports requiring aerobic activity or intermittent activity, where the same modes can progress in complexity to include drills for speed or agility. For resistance training, basic movements can be progressed to more complex multi-joint exercises that challenge stability. For example, a starting point might be a bilateral exercise on a weight machine, with eventual progression to unilateral, dynamic movements with free weights. For sports-specific training with elements such as plyometrics, speed, or agility, general modes can progress to more sports-specific modes as athletes build proficiency. For example, football athletes might progress from linear speed training to sprints that require multiple changes of direction.

Intensity Progression

Progressing exercise intensity is critical to optimizing training outcomes. Progression involves gradual increases in effort. As a general guideline for resistance training, using light to moderate weights (or bodyweight) for 8–15 repetitions is a good starting point. The primary focus should be on proper form and technique to prepare muscles and connective tissues for higher intensities. Intensity for resistance training can be progressed through gradually using heavier loads and lower repetitions once proper technique is established; however, intensity can also be manipulated through other means, like shorter rest times (such as in circuit training), increasing reps and/or sets, or advanced training methods (such as **complex training**, where plyometrics immediately follow high-intensity resistance training). To safely progress intensity, typically only one variable should be changed at a time. For example, an athlete doing 3 sets of 6 squats could progress by increasing the load, adding more reps, doing more sets, or introducing complex training; however, only one of these should be chosen—not all. Limiting intensity increases to 10% or less helps prevent overtraining and injury.

Duration Progression

In general, increases in duration should be limited to 10% or less each week depending on athlete tolerance (i.e., no more than 10% more distance or 10% more time). For resistance training, shorter sessions of 20–30 minutes are an appropriate start, with eventual progression to 45–60 minutes as more exercises, sets, and/or repetitions are included. Heavier weights will also warrant longer durations to account for adequate rest periods. For aerobic training, short sessions of 15–20 minutes are enough to improve fitness in those who are untrained or beginners. As aerobic fitness improves, duration can be gradually increased to 30–60 minutes or longer if athlete goals warrant it. For anaerobic training, performing short intervals with longer rest periods is a good starting point, with progressing either to longer work intervals or shorter rest periods to enhance anaerobic capacity. With flexibility training, the duration of the total stretching time or the duration for each stretch can be progressed. For example, a starting point might be 10 minutes with focus on a few major muscle groups, progressed over time to 20–30-minute sessions with a wider variety of stretches that are held for longer durations.

Periodization Models and Concepts

General Adaptation Syndrome (GAS)

The **general adaptation syndrome (GAS)** theory explains that the body goes through three stages in response to stress. The **alarm phase** is the initial response to a novel or more intense exercise stress, temporarily reducing performance due to soreness or fatigue. The alarm phase can last hours to weeks depending on the nature of the stress. In the **resistance phase**, the body adapts to the stress if it is appropriately applied and structured, returning to normal function or even to improved function and performance (termed **supercompensation**). The **exhaustion phase** occurs when stress continues for too long without adequate recovery, preventing adaptation. An athlete in the exhaustion phase is likely to experience performance decreases, stagnation, and increased fatigue as symptoms of overreaching or overtraining.

The intent of properly structured periodization related to GAS is to maximize supercompensation responses in the resistance phase and avoid athletes entering the exhaustion phase. Avoiding excessive loading, significant variance, and monotony in exercise programs, as well as being attuned to the individual stressors experienced by athletes, will help to promote optimal performance.

Stimulus-Fatigue-Recovery-Adaptation Theory and the Fitness-Fatigue Paradigm

The **stimulus-fatigue-recovery-adaptation** theory posits that a training stimulus or stressor leads to fatigue, which is then followed by a period of recovery that results in an adaptation. This series of stress, fatigue, recovery, and adaptation repeats itself throughout each session or training cycle. In addition, the magnitude of the stressor dictates the extent of the response—for example, a very high training volume will result in more fatigue, requiring more recovery if positive adaptations are going to occur. In the context of periodization, this theory can be used to manage the balance between training and recovery, which can occur in the form of lighter, less intense days. For example, a day of very high training volume may be followed by three sequential light days of training to facilitate recovery and positive adaptations.

The **fitness-fatigue paradigm** suggests that every training stimulus produces both increased fitness and increased fatigue. The more intense the training stimulus, the higher the fitness and fatigue. Conversely, a low-intensity training stimulus will not elicit much fatigue, but it also facilitates only minimal fitness. With application to periodization, the intent is to balance the stimulus so that increased fitness is retained or maximized and fatigue is minimized.

The Hierarchy of Periodization

The specific time periods used in periodization move from having general objectives to more specific objectives, though applicability of each time period depends on the athlete and sport. A **multi-year** or **quadrennial** (4-year) plan is the longest period. An example of a general 4-year objective might be to prepare high school freshmen to be competitive for college athletic scholarships as seniors. The **macrocycle** is the next-longest period, encompassing the entire sport season (from one year, termed an **annual** plan, to several months) and is further divided into preparatory, competitive, and transition periods. Each macrocycle is divided into multiple **mesocycles**, also termed blocks of training, which can last several weeks to several months. Mesocycles typically represent a specific phase of training, such as hypertrophy, strength, or power. **Microcycles** are small training cycles within the mesocycle, such as 1–4 weeks. Within the microcycle are individual training days, where each day may have one (or more) training sessions that can last up to several hours. The training session is the shortest unit of periodization and the most specific, since it contains clearly structured variables like exercises, sets and reps, and rest periods.

Types of Periodization

In **traditional periodization**, the sets and repetitions are maintained at a constant while the training load changes (whether from lighter to heavier or heavier to lighter). For example, a volleyball athlete might progress in gradually heavier loads across 5 sets of 5 back squats in a training cycle and then gradually decrease the load in preparation for competition. It is important to distinguish that while this type of periodization is often termed **linear periodization**, the volume-load is not necessarily linear, making this term inaccurate.

Daily undulating periodization involves significant changes in volume and load from day to day. For example, the same volleyball athlete might have a low-volume, high-load weightlifting day for strength or power and then a high-volume, low-load weightlifting day for endurance the next day, with the intent of developing multiple fitness components throughout the week. Daily undulating periodization is sometimes termed **non-linear periodization**, but this is a less accurate term since traditional periodization is technically non-linear, as described above.

Neither periodization model shows a clear edge in effectiveness for all situations. The choice of model should be based on athlete needs, sport demands, and the timing of the sport season.

Periods in a Periodization Model

The preparatory and first transition period are the first two of the four training periods in a periodization model. The objective of the **preparatory period** is to build a base of training to serve as the foundation for eventual training and competition that is more intense. Of the four periods, this one is often the longest and typically corresponds with the off-season, during which there is no active competition. The preparatory period begins with a **general preparatory phase**, focusing on high volume, low intensity, and general skills to build endurance and hypertrophy. Next, the preparatory period shifts to the **specific preparatory phase**, focusing on more sport-specific movements and gradually increasing intensity and decreasing volume.

The **first transition period** serves as a bridge between the preparatory and competitive periods. This is a shorter period that allows athletes to recover from the preparatory period's high-volume training and prepare for the higher-intensity training of the competitive period. It typically uses a **strength/power phase** with focus on sport-specific training while ramping up intensity that is close to competition levels.

The competitive and second transition periods are the second two of the four training periods in a periodization model. As the name suggests, the **competitive period** is when the main competitions occur. The focus here is on sport-specific techniques and high-intensity, low-volume training to increase strength and power. **Peaking** is a 1–2-week period that may occur during the competitive period, typically coordinated with the most important competition(s). For sports with a longer season, the competitive period may encompass a **maintenance program** that can last for months, where microcycles contain regular variations in volume and intensity to reduce fatigue and prevent overtraining.

The **second transition period**, also known as **restoration** or **active rest,** links the competitive season and the preparatory period. This period typically lasts 1–4 weeks, though it may be longer if injury rehabilitation is needed. During this time for physical and mental recovery, training is low in both volume and intensity and typically is not sport specific. The second transition period is an opportune time for athletes to engage in a variety of cross-training activities to stay physically active without the stressors of intense, sport-specific training.

Individualization

An important key to effective periodization is individualization. While all levels of athletes can benefit from periodization, training programs should account for individual needs and experience levels. With teams that may have a mix of individual needs, varying the periodization plan to avoid one-size-fits-all plans is vital.

Periodization for novice athletes is typically simple, such as using traditional periodization to start with general physical preparedness. The emphasis is on mastering basic skills and developing a broad base of conditioning. Training volume is high, while intensity is low to moderate. Once the athlete has a solid foundation of endurance, strength, and technique, more advanced training methods can be introduced.

Periodization for advanced athletes is typically more complex, often using daily undulating periodization. Since advanced athletes have already developed a strong conditioning base and technical skills, the periodization emphasis is more on optimizing performance for competition.

Programs for Athletes During the Injury/Reconditioning Period

Modifications, Indications, and Contraindications

A **modification** is a change in an aspect of a given exercise. In the context of rehabilitation and reconditioning, the change would typically be to accommodate some type of physical limitation and avoid overstressing healing tissues. For example, an athlete recovering from a shoulder injury might receive a modification to perform wall push-ups rather than push-ups from the ground.

An **indication** is a reason or condition (such as an injury) that requires a given form of treatment or exercise. For example, a track athlete with an ankle injury needs to maintain lower body strength and endurance even if they cannot run. Using an exercise bike could be indicated for aerobic conditioning so they can maintain lower body function without putting pressure on their ankle.

A **contraindication** is a condition or situation that makes an exercise, movement, or treatment inadvisable because it would cause more harm than benefit. For example, the same athlete's injured ankle would contraindicate running, high-impact exercises (such as plyometrics), and agility movements because these movements demand high levels of stability that the recovering tissue is not yet ready to withstand.

Macrotrauma and Microtrauma

Macrotrauma is typically associated with an acute, sudden event that overloads tissue and causes injury. Examples of macrotrauma include fractures (bone), dislocations and subluxations (joints), strains or contusions (muscles), and sprains (ligaments). Additionally, strains and sprains are classified into three degrees by severity, where a first-degree strain or sprain involves a partial tear of some tissues, a second-degree strain or sprain involves a partial tear with weakness and instability, and a third-degree strain or sprain involves a complete tear.

Microtrauma, also known as overuse injury, is the result of repetitive stress applied over extended periods of time rather than a single acute event. Stress fractures are an example of bone microtrauma, and tendonitis is an example of tendon microtrauma. Microtrauma can have various causes, including poor biomechanics or alignment, poor technique, and training errors. For example, a long-distance runner who performs high weekly volumes of running on hard surfaces with poor biomechanics might experience a tibial stress fracture because of the chronic, repetitive impact to the bone.

Phases of Tissue Healing

Tissue healing after an injury occurs in three distinct phases, though the length of each phase can vary depending on the type and severity of the injury.

In the **inflammatory response phase**, which lasts less than a week, the body responds to the injury through releasing various substances to promote tissue healing. Blood vessels dilate to increase blood flow and promote the removal of pathogens. Symptoms during this phase include **edema** (swelling), redness, and pain.

In the **fibroblastic repair phase**, which can begin a few days after injury and last up to 2 months, the healing process promotes improved tissue integrity to the injured area. Scar tissue, collagen fibers, and new capillaries form, creating a foundation for further repair.

In the **maturation-remodeling phase**, the tissue laid down during the previous phase continues to strengthen and heal. This phase can last from months to years. Collagen fibers become stronger through hypertrophy and begin to align, improving their ability to withstand force and stress.

Treatment Goals During Tissue Healing

During the **inflammatory phase**, the main goal is to protect the injured area to avoid disrupting new, healing tissue. Depending on the nature of the injury, some light or unloaded range of motion exercises may be indicated, or the injury may need complete rest. Other uninjured areas should be used to maintain fitness. For example, an athlete with a knee injury can still perform exercises for the upper body, abdominals, and hips.

The goal of the **fibroblastic repair phase** is to continue promoting healing through the right balance of stress on the newly forming collagen fibers without causing pain. Too much stress will prolong healing, but too little stress can limit range of motion. In general, exercises should move through a controlled, pain-free, full range of motion. Submaximal loads of resistance training and slower speeds may be included, as well as exercises for balance and **neuromuscular control** (maintaining joint stability through sensory input).

The goal of the **maturation-remodeling phase** is fully restored function and a return to full activity. Exercises from the previous phase are progressed with gradual loading, along with incorporating sport-specific movements. Returning to full activity should be monitored to ensure the tissue has healed adequately.

Exercise Progression

Progressing exercises through the process of rehabilitation and reconditioning allows the healing tissues to gradually acclimate to increased stress, with the goal of full return to activity. Range of motion is one example of progression where exercises might start in a limited range and progress to full range of movement in each direction at the joint. For example, an athlete with a lateral ankle sprain should initially avoid lateral movement but may eventually progress to standing on a wobble board to enhance balance and promote ankle stability. Strength training progression is a second example. An injured athlete might start with isometric exercises where muscles are contracted without joint movement, then progress to isotonic exercises that move through a full range of motion with light weights and, eventually, heavier weights. A third example is progression from general to sports-specific training with variables such as velocity. For example, the athlete recovering from an ankle sprain who has regained appropriate range of motion and strength might start with low-velocity agility movements. Eventually, they can gradually progress to higher-velocity agility movements that involve quick changes of direction as per the requirements of their sport.

Scope of Practice in Rehabilitation and Reconditioning

The strength and conditioning professional's primary contribution to the rehabilitation and reconditioning process is to understand and apply exercise modalities and exercise techniques to promote athlete recovery. This includes actions like demonstrating correct technique, monitoring progress of the training program, and adjusting the program as needed. Additionally, it is the strength and conditioning professional's responsibility to be informed on factors like type and stage of injury, athlete characteristics, and performance goals in developing programs.

It is not in the scope of practice for a strength and conditioning professional to diagnose or directly treat injuries. Effective injury rehabilitation is done as part of a collaborative team where no single individual fulfills all roles. For example, an athlete who experiences an acute injury may initially receive care from the athletic trainer and get an injury diagnosis from a physician or physical therapist. The work of these other professionals provides guidelines, such as indications and contraindications, to help shape an appropriate and effective program for the athlete, which is created by the strength and conditioning professional.

Exercise Technique

Movement Preparation

Warm-Ups

An effective warm-up needs to provide both physical and psychological preparation for success in the activity. A **general warm-up** consists of aerobic movements that are rhythmic and use large muscle groups (such as most steady-state cardiovascular activities). General warm-ups result in increased heart rate, body temperature, metabolism, and blood flow to working muscles. The **specific warm-up** not only provides further physical preparation but psychological preparation as well through practicing movements and skills that are directly relevant to the sport or activity, allowing the athlete to feel a higher level of success and readiness for the demands of the sport. Dynamic stretches focusing on the muscle groups and ranges of motion to be used are commonly included in the specific warm-up. Another psychological readiness component of the specific warm-up is rehearsing sports-specific skills at lower intensities or speeds. For example, soccer players might practice dribbling the ball and changing direction at slower speeds, or weightlifters might perform drills for their lifts with just an empty bar.

The RAMP Protocol

The RAMP protocol has elements of a general warm-up and specific warm-up but applies more specifically to the demands of a given sport and enhances individual athlete performance through the incorporation of three distinct phases. The first phase, **Raise**, raises body temperature through aerobic movements. The aerobic movements are carefully selected toward improving sports-specific skills and movements. For example, using Raise in a basketball warm-up would go beyond steady-state jogging and might involve aspects like multidirectional jogging. The second phase, **Activation** and **Mobilization**, focuses on activating key muscle groups and enhancing mobility for all needed ranges of motion, such as through dynamic stretching. For example, the basketball warm-up might include lunge walks with overhead reaching and walking knee lifts. The third phase, **Potentiation**, involves the rehearsal of movements at intensities that start low and gradually progress. With the basketball example, athletes might practice passing, dribbling, and shooting at low speeds before increasing their speed to mimic that of real-time gameplay.

Static and Dynamic Stretching

Static stretching involves moving a body segment to a given endpoint and holding the stretch motionless for 15–30 seconds (or more) with the target muscle group relaxed. Static stretching improves range of motion with a relatively low risk of injury because the slow movement stimulates the **Golgi tendon organ**, provoking muscle relaxation, and does not stimulate the **muscle spindle reflex** which would cause the muscle to contract. As an example, a wall stretch for the gastrocnemius and soleus allows the muscles on the back of the lower leg to lengthen as the stretch is held.

Dynamic stretching actively moves a body segment or joint through a functional range of motion. Unlike static stretching, dynamic stretches are not held motionless, so the muscles involved do not fully relax. While dynamic stretching may be less effective at improving flexibility over time, it can be more sports-specific because it can mimic movement patterns and use multiple muscle groups working together. In contrast to the static wall stretch, a dynamic stretch for the gastrocnemius and soleus would be a heel-to-toe walk rolling through a full range of motion at the foot and ankle by exaggerating movements of the gait cycle.

Cues and Precautions for Static Stretching

General cues for static stretching include controlling the speed of the movement, eliciting muscle relaxation responses, and using proper body positioning. Regarding the speed of the movement, an athlete should be advised to slowly move into the static stretch position. Quick movements should be avoided because they can increase injury risk by provoking the muscle to contract via the muscle spindle reflex, as in ballistic stretching. Once the athlete is in the stretch position, they should gradually increase the intensity only to the point of mild discomfort, then hold the stretch for 15–30 seconds (or more). It is important that the athlete breathes and stays as relaxed as possible to elicit optimal relaxation response in the muscle. Stretching should not be performed in areas with acute injury or areas that elicit sensations other than mild discomfort, such as pain or numbness. Static stretching also should not be performed without a short general warm-up to raise body temperature. Good posture and body mechanics should be used to maximize the stretch and best isolate the targeted muscle group. For example, most stretches should be done with the spine straight to maintain stabilization in the rest of the body.

Cues and Precautions for Dynamic Stretching

While dynamic stretching involves movement, it is important to cue that the movement is controlled to reduce injury risk. Dynamic stretching is not about moving body segments as far as possible in their end ranges of motion. Rather, an athlete should only move through a range of motion that they can control the entire time. The end position should be held with no bouncing. In addition, dynamic stretches should progress gradually in speed and/or range of motion. Because dynamic stretches are typically used to mimic sports-specific activities, cues may be used to emphasize body positions. For example, if using the walking over and under stretch, a cue to keep the knees over the toes may be used to facilitate a stable deep squat position without the knees collapsing in.

PNF Stretching

PNF (proprioceptive neuromuscular facilitation) is a method of stretching characterized by using both passive and active muscle contraction in phases. Due to the nature of the active muscle contraction, PNF stretching is often done with a partner who provides resistance to contract against, though some PNF stretches can be done on one's own with assistance from implements like a stretching strap or wall.

While there are multiple types of PNF techniques, each type begins with a passive stretch held for 10 seconds. In **hold-relax**, resistance is then applied for 6 seconds to facilitate isometric muscle contraction, followed by a 30-second passive stretch. In **contract-relax**, the muscle contraction against resistance is concentric rather than isometric and is followed by a 30-second passive stretch. In a **hold-relax with agonist contraction**, the phase after the 10-second passive stretch is the same as hold-relax and then involves a third phase pairing concentric agonist contraction with the assisted passive stretch. This type of PNF is most effective at improving flexibility.

Cues and Precautions for PNF Stretching

Since PNF stretches are often done with a partner, cues and precautions apply to both the individual being stretched and the one assisting. Cues and precautions for the individual being stretched are similar to those of static stretching, like only holding to the point of mild discomfort and maintaining the ability to breathe and relax. Even during the phases of PNF stretching that involve applying force, the individual being stretched should avoid holding their breath. They also need to be clear in communicating when an end-range of motion has been reached so that the person assisting does not force the muscles beyond their stretch capacity.

It is important that the person assisting is clear in providing verbal cues to the individual being stretched. This may include explaining when they are applying resistance through an isometric force and telling the person being stretched how long to contract the muscles and when they can relax. Many assisted PNF stretches require stabilizing other areas of the body, such as keeping the non-stretching leg securely on the ground during a PNF hamstring stretch and keeping the stretching leg straight. Stabilizing force should not be applied directly on a joint but above or below it.

Optimizing Flexibility

There are multiple modifiable factors to consider in optimizing flexibility for individuals or creating flexibility-enhancing programs. Structures like muscle tissue, fascia, and joint capsules can reduce range of motion if they have restrictions. Incorporating techniques like stretching and self-myofascial release can improve range of motion over time. Stretch tolerance and neural control are factors that can be improved over time with flexibility enhancement techniques, with the body becoming more acclimated to mild discomfort at end-ranges of motion. Resistance training complements flexibility training by increasing force development through full ranges of motion.

To best optimize flexibility in program design, frequency, duration, and intensity are necessary considerations. General guidelines include stretching muscles only after they are warm (such as from a general warm-up), holding static stretches for 15–30 seconds to the point of mild discomfort, and performing stretching multiple times per week. In general, stretching longer than 30 seconds is associated with diminishing returns and is not necessary unless specific goals dictate longer stretch durations.

Modifying Warm-Ups and Flexibility Training

While all types of athletes benefit from effective warm-ups and well-structured flexibility training, the nature of these may look quite different across various populations and needs. For example, older adults are often less flexible than younger adults, and males are often less flexible than females. For less flexible populations, modifying stretches to reduce range of motion is one option. Some individuals are hypermobile, and the increased ranges of motion at joints can make them more susceptible to injury. For these individuals, warm-up movements and stretching should have particular focus in improving stability at joints.

It is important that warm-ups and flexibility techniques are assessed relative to the specific demands of the sport or activity. Movements should be chosen to replicate or enhance ranges of motion for the sport based on optimal levels of flexibility for performance. For example, volleyball players need full range of motion for shoulder flexion to spike the ball, so dynamic shoulder flexion movements would logically be a regular part of a warm-up.

Resistance Training Exercise Techniques

Power Exercises

Power exercises use a barbell and apply quick, explosive, multi-joint movements while incorporating spinal loading and stabilization. Some examples of power exercises are the **push press** and **push jerk**, where the bar is forcefully moved from the front rack position at the shoulders to overhead; the **power clean** and **hang power clean**, where the bar is explosively pulled from the ground to the front rack position at the shoulders; and the **power snatch** and **hang power snatch**, where the bar is pulled forcefully from the floor to overhead and received with elbows extended.

Power exercises should not be spotted, as this poses the risk of injury to the athlete and/or the spotter. Rather, a primary safety precaution with power exercises is for the athlete to do them in ample space where the bar can be dropped without danger. Athletes should be instructed in how to drop the bar safely without injuring themselves, which involves moving the opposite way of where the bar is released or dropped. For example, an athlete who misses locking out their elbows on a snatch with the bar behind their head should release the bar and jump forward out of its path.

Spotting

The main responsibility of the spotter is to keep the athlete safe without compromising their own personal safety. Most barbell exercises should be performed in a power rack to enhance athlete safety by providing a stable place to initiate and return the lift. The only exceptions are power exercises, like the Olympic lifts, which should neither be performed in a rack nor spotted. Spotters for barbell exercises should match or exceed the height and strength of the athlete lifting. Some situations require having more than one spotter, such as with loads that are heavier than a single person could safely spot.

In general, spotters should maintain a wide, stable base of support and a neutral spine. Different exercises may require different spotting grips or body sites. For example, a bench press should be spotted with a narrow, alternated grip, and most upper body dumbbell exercises should be spotted at the wrists. The spotter and athlete must communicate on elements like **liftoff** (moving the bar to the starting position), when the spotter should get involved, and how much spotting assistance is required.

Breathing during Weight Training

In general, athletes should be cued to inhale on the less strenuous phase of the exercise and to exhale through the most strenuous phase, the **sticking point**. For example, the sticking point in a back squat occurs in rising after the descent. The sticking point in a bench press occurs while pressing the bar back up after the descent.

The **Valsalva maneuver** helps maintain spinal position and support during exertion by increasing intra-abdominal pressure with a closed glottis. It is typically used by more experienced athletes during structural exercises that load the spine (such as barbell squats) and where the load is greater than 80% (such as in a 1-repetition maximum). While effective, the Valsalva maneuver carries risks. The brief rise in blood pressure can put more stress on the heart, which can cause dizziness and blackouts. Anyone with existing cardiovascular conditions should not use the Valsalva maneuver in weightlifting. Athletes can maintain spinal support using proper technique and breathing without the need for the Valsalva maneuver, so it is not necessary to use with submaximal loads or less experienced athletes.

Body Position and Form with Free Weight Training

The foundation of almost all weightlifting movements is a **neutral spine**, where the natural curves of the spine are maintained, including a slight **lordotic curve** at the lumbar spine (as opposed to rounding the low back). A neutral spine should be established before lifting the weight and should be maintained throughout the movement. Weight belts can help prevent low back injury in heavy lifts, but, otherwise, the body's core musculature alone should be sufficient to stabilize the spine.

For standing movements, a typical stable stance has the feet slightly outside the hips. For seated or supine movements, stability is created through the **five-point body contact position** in which both feet are flat and the buttocks, shoulders, upper back, and head are firmly planted on a surface. In general, free weight movements should be performed at controlled speeds that reach full ranges of motion. While there are some explosive weightlifting exercises, like the Olympic lifts, control and technique should never be sacrificed for speed.

Various free weight exercises require different types of grips. Without extensively detailing all free weight movements, the most common grips are **pronated** (palms down) and **supinated** (palms up). Proper grip and proper grip width help provide a stable position and prevent injury.

Resistance Machines

Both resistance machines and free weights can be used to apply external load to muscles for goals such as muscular endurance, hypertrophy, or strength, but free weights are more suitable in many situations. Free weight movements have more opportunity to recruit muscles that stabilize posture and work multiple joints. This provides a greater training stimulus and is more applicable to real-life functional movements and sports-specific movements; however, free weight movements are more challenging to perform correctly and may require a spotter for safe execution.

Resistance machines are well-suited when safety or muscle isolation is a main goal. Without freely moving weights, there is a much lower risk of injury, and no spotter is needed. These qualities make resistance machines useful for populations where balance and stability might be an issue, such as older adults or those new to exercise. Resistance machines are also commonly used in hypertrophy goals, such as targeting specific muscle groups to enhance their muscular definition; however, components of resistance machines may need to be adjusted based on individual differences like height or limb length, and they may not fit the dimensions and body types of all individuals.

Body Position and Form with Resistance Machines

Some general considerations for resistance machines overlap with considerations for resistance training in general, including using free weights. For example, movements should typically start with a neutral spine and maintain the position throughout exercise while moving in a slow and controlled manner. While not all resistance machines allow a full range of motion at all joints, going through the greatest ROM possible is typically desirable.

Movements should also be performed with a stable body position throughout the movement where non-working muscle groups and joints remain still. For example, in a low pulley seated row, the torso should remain upright without jerking or leaning back as the arms execute the backward movement. Joints at full extension should maintain a slight bend, such as avoiding knee lockout in the hip sled (leg press) machine.

Many resistance training machines have points of contact for stability, like seats and back pads, as well as pads for minimizing unwanted movement, such as the leg pads on an abdominal crunch machine. Seats, pads, and/or handles may need to be adjusted in line with the manufacturer's directions and based on the user's height or body size.

Core Stability Training

The **core** is not limited to just the abdominal muscles but also involves muscles that support the axial skeleton and function to transfer force to the limbs. The core is often trained through isolation exercises and/or instability-based exercises. Core isolation exercises are typically ones that flex, extend, laterally flex, or rotate the spine, such as abdominal crunches. Instability-based exercises are ones done on an unstable surface, such as stability ball rollouts or standing on a wobble board.

Core isolation and instability exercises can be useful for specific injury prevention or rehabilitation, novice exercisers, or for targeting spinal stability specifically; however, since the body's core naturally works synergistically with other muscle groups, the real-life application of isolated core movements is limited. In addition, instability-based training reduces the amount of force the body can develop, so it is not particularly useful for goals of enhancing strength and power. Therefore, training the core through enhancing its function and stability has the most sports-specific application when multi-joint, free weight movements are used rather than isolation or instability-based movements.

Bodyweight Exercises

Bodyweight exercises don't involve external resistance. Only the weight of the body is used. **Calisthenics** is another name for bodyweight exercises done rhythmically or repeatedly to build strength and improve fitness. Common calisthenics movements include variations of pull-ups, push-ups, dips, and squats (often single-leg variations, like pistol squats). A main advantage of bodyweight exercises is that they are portable and inexpensive. Only a small space is needed for many bodyweight movements, and many do not require any equipment at all (though there are some bodyweight movements that require an apparatus like a bar, such as pull-ups or dips). As another advantage, most bodyweight movements use multiple muscle groups, promoting core stability since they are not isolating a single muscle group. Also, most bodyweight movements can be easily modified for different fitness levels, goals, and abilities.

The main disadvantage of bodyweight movements is that they are not ideal for improving absolute strength. With the use of only bodyweight, an athlete can eventually encounter a plateau since there is no external resistance to add. While increasing the intensity of bodyweight exercises can be done through changing the exercise or the body's positioning, building absolute strength is better done through resistance machines or free weight training.

Strongman Training

Strongman training uses weighted objects that are often of irregular size and weight, such as tires and logs. While some of the movements and lifts may look similar to those of free weight barbell movements, strongman movements often require generating strength from a wider variety of body positions and stances. Since techniques may differ based on the shape, size, and object, strongman training can provide a greater variety and stability challenge than traditional free weights; however, the stability challenge typically means that an athlete will not be able to do the same weight with a strongman implement compared to using a barbell.

Considerations for proper technique in strongman training have overlap with those of free weight movements. For example, flipping a tire properly has similarities to a deadlift, including the use of a conventional or sumo deadlift stance and keeping the hips below the shoulders to use the body's leverage effectively and avoid low back injury. The log clean and press has similarities to a clean and jerk, such as maintaining a neutral spine throughout the first and second pull and forcefully driving the log overhead through extending at the elbows, knees, and hips.

Kettlebell Training

Kettlebells are round implements with a handle that permit movements like swinging and pressing. Fitness kettlebells are made of cast iron. The size of fitness kettlebells increases along with their weight, and they tend to be more common in fitness facilities. Competition kettlebells are made of steel and are the same size regardless of weight. Kettlebells are more portable and versatile than a modality like resistance machines, so they can be an effective implement for small spaces or larger groups of athletes. In addition, using kettlebells can improve cardiovascular fitness and muscular fitness simultaneously. For example, repeated bouts of a dynamic exercise like the **kettlebell swing** can maintain an elevated heart rate at the same time as strengthening muscles of core stability and hip extension; however, for sport-specific goals like improving strength or power, modalities like dumbbell workouts are more effective. Similarly, specific cardiovascular fitness goals like improving aerobic endurance or anaerobic efficiency are targeted more effectively through movements like running or sprint intervals than kettlebell exercises.

Olympic Weightlifting and Plyometric Exercise Techniques

Preparatory Position for the Olympic Lifts

There are two **Olympic lifts**—the clean and jerk and the snatch. In a strength and conditioning context with goals such as improving power and force production, athletes may do these lifts or elements or derivatives of these lifts, such as hang cleans, hang snatches, and push jerks.

Olympic lifts require an Olympic-style barbell and Olympic-style weight plates. The barbell's rotating sleeves allow the weight to move freely during the lift, reducing injury risk and improving efficiency, and Olympic plates can be dropped without damage. The athlete should have adequate space and stable flooring to drop the barbell safely if needed. The Olympic lifts are often done on weightlifting platforms that provide ideal traction and bounce.

Both lifts start with pulling the bar from the floor. The setups for the clean and jerk and the snatch have many similarities. Both begin with the feet flat on the floor, weight in the midfoot, a neutral or slightly arched spine, the head in line with the spine, the gaze straight ahead or slightly up, the shoulder blades back and down to engage the latissimus dorsi muscles, pronated or hook grip, and the shoulders slightly over the bar. The main difference in setup is the grip width. A snatch involves a wider grip than the clean.

Preparatory Position for Power Exercises Involving Pressing Overhead

Both the **push press** and **push jerk** start at the shoulders (often called the **front rack position**, where the bar is 'racked' on the shoulders in front.) These lifts can be done from a power rack or from doing a clean from the floor and finishing in the front rack. If taking the lifts from a power rack, the rack supports should be at shoulder level so that the athlete can properly step under the bar for positioning. The athlete holds the bar with a pronated grip that is slightly wider than the shoulders with the chest tall and elbows lifted (though the extent of elbow lift depends on various individual factors of the athlete). The feet should be about hip-width apart with the knees and toes slightly pointed out. The preparatory dip phase is similar in both movements—the athlete descends no deeper than a quarter squat by initiating hip and knee flexion while keeping the torso upright and the feet flat. The main difference between the push press and push jerk is the ending catch position. The push press is caught with full knee and hip extension, while the push jerk is caught with knee and hip flexion.

The Power Clean

The **power clean** begins with the barbell on the floor and the athlete's grip slightly wider than shoulder-width. The first pull describes the movement of the bar from the floor to the knees. In this first pull, the shoulders and hips rise at the same time, the bar remains close to the shins, and the hips and knees begin to extend but do not yet reach full extension. The transition marks the shift where the bar is accelerated more explosively once it passes the knees and the knees move back to make way for the bar's rapid ascent. The second pull involves **triple extension**, where the hips, knees, and ankles simultaneously extend, the arms remain straight, the shoulders shrug upward, and the lifter may move with enough force to briefly leave the ground. The catch immediately follows the second pull. During the catch, the athlete rapidly descends under the barbell, rotating the arms around to receive the bar at collarbone height in the front rack position with the torso erect and the hips and knees in slight flexion (in contrast, in the non-power version of the clean, the athlete catches the barbell while in a squat position). In the end position, the athlete stands fully by straightening the legs while keeping the bar in the front rack with elbows high.

THE POWER SNATCH

The **power snatch** begins with the barbell on the floor. The athlete's grip should be wider than a clean grip. Appropriate grip width depends on the athlete's body size and limb length and can be measured from the edge of a clenched fist to the opposite shoulder with the arm extended laterally or by the distance from each elbow when the arms are out to the sides. In the first pull, the bar moves from floor to knee height through extension of the hips and knees while maintaining a neutral spine, a constant torso angle, and extended elbows. In the transition, the hips explosively extend to generate power and accelerate the bar upward. The bar will typically make contact high on the thighs. The **triple extension** of the second pull is marked by hip, knee, and ankle extension. The athlete should maintain straight elbows as the shoulders shrug upward, and the athlete may leave the ground briefly. The catch for the snatch is performed by rapidly descending under the barbell to receive it overhead in full elbow extension with slightly flexed hips and knees (in contrast, the catch for the non-power version of the snatch is performed in a squat position). The movement ends by standing fully and extending the hips and knees while stabilizing the bar's overhead position.

CORRECTIONS AND MODIFICATIONS OF TECHNIQUE IN THE OLYMPIC LIFTS

The Olympic lifts are both highly technical lifts that require rapid changes in force production. In addition to strength and power, accurate technique is critical to achieve the most effective positions of the body and the barbell. Without providing an exhaustive list of all technique errors, common corrections include ones that target balance, body position, and timing. For example, if an athlete begins with their shoulders too far behind the bar, their balance shifts backward and triple extension in the second pull will be reduced, which also reduces the amount of acceleration applied to the bar. Other common errors include bending the arms prematurely before the body has reached triple extension or receiving the bar in a poor catch position that lacks stability. **Part practice** exercises can be used for portions of the Olympic lifts that need correction or modification. For example, the Romanian deadlift (RDL) helps to reinforce proper position for the transition phase. The hang power clean or hang power snatch help reinforce posture and balance, especially in the second pull. The push jerk (or snatch grip push jerk) helps reinforce proper catch position with elbows in full extension.

Speed, Agility, and Plyometric Techniques

STARTING POSITION FOR SPRINTING

There is no single best body position for sprinting, as it will depend on the nature of the athlete's sport. For example, track athletes performing dedicated sprinting events will start with their feet in blocks and either both hands (4-point staggered start) or one hand (3-point staggered start) touching the ground. Other types of athletes may need to execute sprints from a standing position (2-point stance) in multiple directions, such as in soccer, baseball, or basketball.

The following general aspects hold true for body positioning for sprinting in most sports and activities. A staggered stance, with feet about shoulder-width apart and the dominant leg in front, is typically the most effective stance to initiate acceleration. Body weight should be shifted so that the front leg is bearing more weight and the center of gravity is over the front foot. The front leg should have about a 90-degree bend. While the back leg will be first to move at the initiation of sprinting, both legs will generate explosive force simultaneously.

THE CROUCHED START (2-POINT STANCE)

The **crouched start** is a 2-point stance that allows athletes to initiate acceleration for sprinting. Unlike a 3-point or 4-point stance, where an athlete has one or both hands on the ground (commonly used for sprint events in track), the 2-point stance of the crouched start has only the feet in contact with the ground, making it generally applicable for many sports. The athlete begins in a staggered stance with the dominant leg forward and the back leg about 1–2 foot-lengths behind, though the distance between the legs can vary depending on the individual. The back knee is flexed, bringing the shin closer to the ground, and body weight should shift forward so that the front leg bears slightly more weight. The center of gravity should be over the front foot. The arm opposite the front leg should be raised with an elbow bend that places the hand at about forehead-height. The other arm is pulled back with a bend at the elbow and the hand at about hip level. In this position, the athlete is now ready to effectively apply force to the ground through the legs with assistance from the arms.

3-POINT OR 4-POINT START

An athlete using a 3-point or 4-point stance has both feet and one or both hands on the ground and may or may not use blocks depending on the nature of the activity. While there may be some slight variations in posture, there are some general guidelines for these body positions. The hips should be higher than the shoulders, and the feet should be about 2 foot-lengths apart. The shin of the back leg should be closer to parallel with the ground than vertical. If the hips are too high, the body weight may shift forward, placing more weight on the hands and limiting assistance of the arms in initiating the sprint. The athlete should maintain a neutral posture with the head and neck in line with the spine. If the athlete shows a break in posture by hyperextending the neck, this may cause an undesirable early lift of the torso, reducing the acceleration that can be applied.

APPLICATION OF FORCE TO SPRINT TECHNIQUE

Force is the product of **mass** and **acceleration**. Successful speed or sprint technique requires the athlete to move their body mass at a high rate of acceleration through the production of force. An athlete who can rapidly apply large amounts of force will be more successful at sprinting. Training for optimal execution of sprint technique needs to focus on two factors related to force. The first is the **rate of force development (RFD)**, or the extent of maximal force development in a minimal time, often conceptualized as explosive strength. The second factor is **impulse**, which is the extent to which momentum changes. Force is applied through impulse every time the athlete's feet touch the ground while sprinting.

To improve speed in sprint technique, an athlete will need to apply forces at a greater rate. This can be done through using optimal stride length and stride frequency. Stride length depends on the individual, so there is no single best length. Working within an athlete's natural gait cycle is typically best, since over-striding can create a slower pace and increase forces placed on the body, leading to increased injury risk. For stride frequency, emphasizing explosive strength will reduce ground contact time, thus improving speed.

THE STRETCH-SHORTENING CYCLE AND SPRINT/SPEED TECHNIQUE

The **stretch-shortening cycle** describes how muscles contract explosively to reach maximal force in minimal time. It is used in movements with rapid changes in velocity, such as plyometrics and sprinting, and can be conceptualized as an elastic band or a coiled spring. The stretch-shortening cycle is present in the gait cycle as an eccentric contraction during the feet touching down and a concentric contraction as the feet leave the ground. The **amortization phase** is the phase in between the eccentric and concentric contraction.

The principle of the stretch-shortening cycle is applied with techniques to minimize ground contact time in sprinting, contributing to greater speeds. When the eccentric contraction portion is rapid and the amortization phase is kept short, the stored elastic energy of the muscles is stimulated, causing a more forceful concentric contraction. In addition, applying optimal amounts of force in sprinting is an application of the stretch-shortening cycle, as loading the muscles and tendons allows them to recoil like a spring, enhancing explosive movement that benefits speed.

Optimal Sprint Technique at Acceleration and Maximal Velocity

The phase of **acceleration** occurs immediately after starting a sprint and is the time from when the athlete leaves the blocks or starting line until they reach maximal velocity. The stride length initially will appear short compared to the longer stride length utilized when the athlete reaches maximal velocity. The feet are dorsiflexed to enhance propulsive force into the ground for continued acceleration. The head should remain in line with the spine. The torso should remain angled slightly forward with the athlete's gaze toward the ground. As the athlete increases in acceleration and begins to reach maximal velocity, the torso and head should rise at the same rate. Once the athlete is at **maximal velocity**, the athlete's posture is upright and vertical with the shoulders over the hips and the athlete's gaze straight ahead. The shoulders are relaxed, and the arm swings occur at the same rate as the legs in each gait cycle. The stride rate and stride length are at their peak during maximal velocity to minimize ground contact time and maximize force applied to the ground with each step.

Corrections for Arm Movement Errors

Arm movement technique is a critical part of sprinting effectively since the arm swings assist the legs in their propulsive movement forward. One common error is the arm swings being too short and tight. This can be caused by the athlete holding excess tension in the upper body. The shoulders should remain down and relaxed rather than shrugged upward, and the hands should be relaxed rather than stiff or in tightly clenched fists. Another correction for ineffective arm swing range of motion is to emphasize driving the elbow down and back with the hand going below the line of the waist. Proper arm swing can be practiced with drills such as isolating the arm swing from the leg movement or A-skips.

Another common arm movement error is that the arms have unnecessary extra movement into the transverse plane, crossing the body rather than driving linearly. This reduces speed and efficiency because the body must use extra energy to counterbalance. Similar to correcting for excessively short and tight arm swings, the correction to drive the elbow down and back can be effective, as well as cueing to keep the elbows close to the body.

Corrections or Modifications for Decreased Mobility

The primary mobility need for sprinters is lower body mobility, specifically mobility in the muscles that stabilize the pelvis and the muscles of the legs. The pelvis is stabilized by four groups of muscles—the abdominals, low back muscles, hip extensors, and hip flexors. Lacking appropriate mobility in the hip flexors can pull the pelvis out of alignment into an **anterior pelvic tilt**. Having some degree of anterior tilt is natural and may not be an issue unless it is excessive and limiting the athlete's hip extension. In this case, the athlete would benefit from mobility techniques like self-myofascial release, stretching for the hip flexors, and training the abdominals and hip extensors to build strength and stabilization for the pelvis.

Focusing on hamstrings is particularly beneficial for sprint athletes, especially for those experiencing chronic pain or tightness. In the gait cycle of sprinting, the hamstring of the back leg contracts eccentrically under load. This can overload the hamstrings beyond their capacity, causing injury. Ankle mobility is also important for effective dorsiflexion when sprinting. Tight calf muscles can limit ankle mobility. Regular mobility techniques like self-myofascial release and stretching are beneficial for these lower body muscle groups.

Corrections for Lower Body Errors

Over-striding and **under-striding** are two common lower body technique errors in sprinting. While stride length has individual variance, over-striding can be seen when an athlete's foot lands too far in front of the body. Athletes may over-stride to increase their speed as a compensation for lower stride frequency. Cueing to have the foot land slightly in front of the body and having the athlete try a higher stride frequency are two corrections for over-striding. The fast feet drill can be helpful in emphasizing stride frequency.

With under-striding, steps that are too short limit the body's ability to apply force into the ground. The athlete can be cued to push off the ground more forcefully, reaching triple extension at the hip, knee, and ankle of the back leg and having the front knee's leg higher—up to 80 degrees. If the athlete's under-striding is primarily due to a lack of knee drive, strengthening the muscles that flex the hip can be beneficial. In addition, the A-skip drill can be used to emphasize force production in under-striding.

Starting Position for Agility Techniques

Starting positions for agility techniques depend on the nature of the sport. In general, agility movements that start from a stationary body position should use an **athletic ready position**, with a stance slightly wider than the hips or shoulders, the knees slightly bent, and the spine and head in a neutral position. Both feet are fully in contact with the ground, and the center of gravity is shifted slightly forward. This athletic ready position best prepares the body to go from stationary to producing force and explosiveness.

Other sports require **reactive agility**, or the ability to change body positions in response to a real-time, unplanned stimulus. In these scenarios, the athlete may be already sprinting or running. The stance or base of support should be wide enough to change direction or speed quickly without compromising balance. There should also be some degree of hip, knee, and ankle flexion. The athlete should initiate any changes of direction through the trunk and hips, and the legs will immediately follow.

Body Positioning in Executing Agility Techniques

Many sport-specific agility scenarios are inherently unpredictable, and there are a wide variety of directional movements that can occur during many sports; however, there are some general guidelines for visual focus, body position, and action of the limbs. Visually focusing on an opponent's trunk, shoulders, and hips will help the athlete anticipate their next move and react quickly. Proper body positioning includes orienting the trunk and hips toward the desired direction of travel to increase acceleration, leaning forward during acceleration to maximize force development, and keeping a lower center of mass when starting or ending changes of direction. With limb movement, proper positioning of both the arms and the legs is important. If possible, arms should swing powerfully to enhance force production through the lower body (while understanding that the arms may need to be used otherwise for actions like intercepting or blocking). Leg action while moving should accentuate pushing the ground away for maximal force development, and leg action while braking should involve flexion at the hips, knees, and ankles.

Body Position in Initiating Braking

Braking is decelerating the body. In agility techniques, braking effectively is critical to change directions efficiently and to reduce injury. At the lower body, **triple flexion** is used to initiate braking, where flexing at the hips, knees, and ankles helps to absorb force. In addition, the knees should remain aligned over the ankles rather than moving inward to adduction, as this can overload the knees and increase the risk of injury. At the torso, the athlete's posture becomes more upright to move the center of gravity higher and decrease momentum. The arms will decrease their range of motion, as shorter arm swings assist in deceleration. The body weight should be closer to the heels than the toes, as this will increase ground contact time and further assist in braking.

Neurophysiological Considerations for Agility Techniques

Agility is defined as the combined use of change of direction ability and perceptual-cognitive ability. In many sport-specific situations, it is not enough to be able to change directions through applying force. Rather, the demands require rapid response to an unpredictable stimulus, such as running toward the path of the ball in basketball as it is passed and dribbled by the opposing team. These types of requirements are **neurophysiological** requirements, where the brain, nervous system, and muscles work together.

The response time of an athlete can be affected by these perceptual-cognitive demands of agility. For example, in many sports, like football or basketball, an athlete has only a limited time to change directions quickly to successfully intercept the ball. Therefore, agility technique should incorporate elements of perceptual-cognitive training that are relevant to the sport. Specific elements may include reaction time, accuracy, decision-making, situational awareness, anticipation, visual scanning, and pattern recognition. For example, a coach may incorporate stimuli like a light, audible signal, pointing, or throwing a ball to increase perceptual-cognitive stress that will simulate sport-specific situations.

Methods for Developing Effective Agility Techniques

Effective agility techniques rely on strength, change of direction ability, and perceptual-cognitive ability.

Strength requirements are similar for agility and speed since both require considerable amounts of force production to change the body's velocity. For the best application of specificity, weightlifting exercises and movements should have elements of both speed and strength. For example, Olympic lifts and their variations require considerable amounts of power and force production and would be preferable over weight machines in developing strength for agility.

Since agility is comprised of both change of direction ability and perceptual-cognitive ability, developing both is vital to improving agility performance. Incorporating change of direction drills based on sports-specific needs should be a regular part of training. These drills should be gradually progressed to continue challenging athletes. Perceptual-cognitive ability training can be incorporated into agility drills with elements such as anticipation, accuracy, and quick decision-making. For example, elements of uncertainty, like an audible signal, can be incorporated into a change of direction drill.

Braking and Deceleration

The principles for braking in agility technique are similar to those in speed technique. Since moving at high velocities requires large amounts of force production, high demands are placed on the body to absorb those forces effectively while decelerating.

Eccentric strength is required to brake effectively and should be included in agility training. An eccentric contraction involves forcible lengthening of the muscle and requires different motor unit recruitment than a concentric contraction. Examples of eccentric strength training techniques include absorbing force in drop landings, lifting weight with two limbs and lowering with one limb, or executing an explosive concentric contraction followed by a slow tempo on the eccentric portion.

Enhancing braking can also be done through **deceleration drills**, where the athlete accelerates rapidly and then decelerates in a controlled manner. In general, athletes should absorb forces with the torso upright and the hips, knees, and ankles all in flexion, and the feet should land in front of the hips. Deceleration drills can be progressed to become more difficult by increasing the speed of acceleration to top speed, requiring a minimal number of steps to decelerate, and/or decelerating in a different direction.

Monitoring and Assessing Agility Development

In a basic sense, agility development can be assessed by monitoring the change in the time it takes an athlete to complete a given drill. For example, an athlete who attains a faster time on the Z-drill after months of training may appear to have developed their agility; however, it is possible that the athlete in question just got faster at running and maintained the same level of agility. Therefore, measuring only time does not account for the perceptual-cognitive and change of direction aspects of agility.

Other ways to monitor agility development besides time include change of direction deficit, ground contact time, entry and exit velocity, and decision-making time. Some of these elements, like velocity, are best measured with high-speed cameras, but others could be measured with simple timing devices. For example, the seconds elapsed between a stimulus and an athlete's decision to move could be measured over time, where fewer seconds elapsed and greater accuracy in movement would indicate that the athlete's perceptual-cognitive quality of agility has improved.

Modifying and Progressing Agility Development

Strength is a significant requirement of sound agility technique and should be a foundational focus for novice athletes. Using dynamic strength movements through multidirectional bodyweight exercises will build strength and improve mobility with low injury risk. Novice athletes can also focus on concentric and eccentric strength, such as with box jumps or drop landings. In transferring agility development to a sports-specific context through drills, novice athletes will benefit from starting with low-intensity plyometrics, acceleration and deceleration, multidirectional movement at low velocities, and drills with simple elements of reaction.

While there is no specific guideline on when an athlete is no longer considered novice and is now advanced, athletes should show proficiency in body positioning, simple agility techniques, and have a base level of consistent strength work before doing more demanding progressions. Advanced athletes can use more technically complex, explosive movements for strength and plyometrics, such as Olympic lifts, loaded jumps, and depth jumps. For drills in sports-specific contexts, advanced athletes can be challenged through faster velocities (such as decelerating from top speed), more aggressive changes of direction, and manipulating space or time constraints (such as timed agility tests).

Change of Direction, Maneuverability, and Agility

Change of direction training for novice athletes can begin with basic movement patterns in various directions at low speeds and decelerating from moderate speeds. Intermediate athletes can progress to decelerating from different directions besides forward, moving at higher velocities as they change directions, and changing directions at cutting angles of 75° or less. Advanced athletes can be challenged with deceleration in all directions and at varying velocities and steep cutting angles of 75° or greater.

Maneuverability is using multiple ways of changing direction in a single drill or scenario, such as shuffling laterally and then running backwards. Novice and intermediate athletes should focus on maintaining efficient body positions. For more advanced athletes, the quick transition in changes of direction while maintaining body position is the focus, such as completing trials of the T-test with the objective of improving their time.

In progressing agility, novice athletes should show competence in the above elements before dedicated agility work and its perceptual-cognitive demands are introduced. Agility drills with simple, limited stimuli can be used for intermediate athletes. Greater levels of cognitive uncertainty can be used for advanced athletes to best mimic real-life sport.

Preparatory Position for Lower Body Plyometric Exercises

Lower body **plyometric exercises** include types of jumps, hops, and bounds where an athlete produces a large amount of force in a short amount of time. The intensity of these movements can vary depending on the number of repetitions, speed, height, and/or changes in direction; however, regardless of the intensity, the general setup for lower body plyometric exercises is typically similar (and the finishing position is often similar to the starting position). The center of gravity should be over the body's base of support. In a standing posture, the center of gravity is just below the navel, so this should be evenly between the two feet as the base of support. The shoulders, knees, and toes should all be in alignment with the hips, ankles, and knees in flexion, though the level of flexion depends on the type of exercise (for example, a squat jump has more flexion than a hop). The knees should remain over the first and second toes in the frontal plane. Knees that are not in this alignment and angled inward (termed **valgus** knees) can put excess stress on the knee joint and increase the risk of injury.

The Stretch-Shortening Cycle in Plyometric Movements

Plyometric movements are marked by their characteristic of using the **stretch-shortening cycle**, where muscles reach maximal force in a short period through quick, explosive movement. Examples of plyometric movements include jumps, hops, and bounds for the lower body and passes, throws, and explosive push-ups for the upper body. The first phase of the stretch-shortening cycle is the **eccentric phase**, where the agonist muscles store energy through being stretched. In a chest pass, for example, this is where the ball is caught as the elbows bend. The second phase is the **amortization phase**, which is a pause before initiating the concentric movement. For plyometric movements, this must be kept short to maximize power production. In a chest pass, there is a very brief pause before throwing the ball back, but if the athlete pauses longer in holding the ball, power production is reduced because the extra time reduces the amount of stored energy. The third phase is the **concentric phase**, where rapid muscle contraction causes powerful movement. In the case of the chest pass, this is when the ball is forcefully thrown back.

Modifications of Lower Body Plyometric Drills

There are four main factors that affect the intensity of lower body plyometric drills. **Points of contact** can be modified to increase or decrease intensity. For example, single-leg movements are more intense than movements that involve using both legs at once. Drills performed at higher **speeds** require more rapid muscle contraction and are more intense than those performed at lower speeds. Drills that involve greater **heights** are more intense due to higher landing forces. **Weight** (whether based on the athlete's weight or externally added weight like a vest) increases intensity since more mass must be moved rapidly. Based on these four factors, intensity can be increased or decreased depending on the athlete's needs and skills. For example, newer athletes who demonstrate proficiency in lower-intensity movements like skipping could progress to drills involving greater heights or speeds.

Volume in plyometric drills is measured as repetitions and sets and can be quantified by distance or the number of foot contacts. Volume and intensity should have an inverse relationship (i.e., more intense drills should be done at lower volumes). For example, a single-leg depth jump is one of the highest intensity lower body plyometric drills, so the volume of these should be kept small to preserve the quality of movement and prevent injury.

Safety Considerations for Plyometric Exercises

Plyometric exercises are effective for increasing power and muscle force production but are not one-size-fits-all and require careful consideration for implementing them in a program. First, there are populations where certain plyometric exercises may be unsafe. Youths whose bones are still developing should not perform high-intensity plyometrics due to the risk of growth plate injuries. Older adults and those with preexisting joint conditions or past injuries should use lower intensity and lower volumes of plyometrics, with further modification or regression if chronic pain is experienced. Athletes with a body weight over 220 lb (100 kg) can experience more force on their joints and higher injury risk with plyometrics and should use lower intensities and lower volumes.

Athletes must have a prerequisite base of strength, technique, and balance. For example, athletes who have not learned how to land properly without valgus knees require more supplemental strengthening before progressing to plyometrics. If an athlete lacks single-leg static balance, they need to improve balance before progressing to dynamic movements like single-leg plyometric drills.

Energy Systems Development

Improving the Lactate Threshold

The **lactate threshold** is the highest exercise intensity that can be maintained before blood lactate significantly increases. Lactate threshold is a desirable aspect to improve for aerobic endurance athletes because it means that they can sustain higher intensities of exercise for longer durations. Training at or above the lactate threshold allows the body to improve its ability to buffer and clear lactate from the blood.

The most accurate way to find an athlete's lactate threshold is in a lab environment. In this lab test, the athlete exercises at progressively higher intensities while blood samples are taken regularly and assessed for lactate levels. Alternatively, lactate threshold can be estimated through field testing with heart rate calculations. In this test, the athlete does 30 minutes of aerobic activity at the highest intensity they can sustain.

Once an athlete has measured or estimated their lactate threshold, training for improvement will require training at or above intensities of the lactate threshold. Depending on the athlete's needs and nature of the sport, this may require different modalities (running, cycling, etc.) and may be done with longer-duration, steady-state exercise at the lactate threshold or shorter, higher-intensity intervals that are above the lactate threshold.

Monitoring Intensity

Using METs and RPE Scales

One **metabolic equivalent (MET)** is equal to the oxygen cost required by the body at rest. An activity that is 5 METs, for example, requires five times as much oxygen than at rest. Most common physical activities have assigned MET values based on research and are often broadly categorized as moderate intensity (3–6 METs) or vigorous intensity (6+ METs). METs can be used to ensure an athlete is working at the appropriate intensity to meet their goals and needs. For example, if an athlete needs to work at a moderate intensity for a recovery day, a corresponding moderate intensity MET activity should be selected to facilitate that recovery.

Rating of perceived exertion (RPE) scales allow athletes to self-rate their exercise intensity. The most common RPE scale is from 1 to 10, where 1 is doing no exercise at all and 10 is a maximal effort. RPE scales can provide a comprehensive scope of how hard an athlete feels they are working since RPE takes multiple factors into account, such as heart rate, breathing rate, fatigue, and others. Like METs, RPE scales can be used to ensure an athlete is staying within the prescribed intensities for their goals and needs.

Using Heart Rate Methods

Heart rate reserve (HRR) is the difference between an athlete's maximal heart rate and their resting heart rate. To ensure the highest accuracy, HRR can be determined through VO_2 max testing or lactate threshold testing where a given percentage of the HRR is used to prescribe and monitor intensity.

In the absence of direct testing, the **Karvonen method** uses an estimated HRR for use in calculating an intensity range. The calculation starts with subtracting the athlete's age from 220 and then subtracting their resting heart rate from the resulting number. This number is multiplied by the desired exercise intensities to provide a range, and the resting heart rate is added back in to the two values used to calculate the intensity range.

Percentage of maximal heart rate begins with subtracting the athlete's age from 220, resulting in an age-predicted maximum heart rate. This number is then multiplied by the desired exercise intensities to yield a range. While this is a quick method, it can have a considerable margin of error since it does not take other factors into account, like the athlete's fitness level.

LSD and Tempo Training

Long, slow distance (LSD) is training done at intensities where the athlete is still able to talk, about 80% of maximal heart rate or 70% of VO_2 max. LSD is slower and longer in duration than an athlete's target race pace and duration. For example, an athlete who normally does a 10-kilometer race in 40 minutes runs just under 6 minutes and 30 seconds per mile. LSD may be prescribed as running at a pace 1–2 minutes slower for 60 minutes. Using LSD can improve aerobic adaptations, such as sparing glycogen, using fat for fuel, and enhancing the oxygen uptake of the muscles; however, it should not be used exclusively, as it does not provide overloading at higher intensities, which an athlete would need to improve their pace.

Tempo training, also called **pace training** or **threshold training**, is done at an intensity at, or slightly greater than, race pace. Tempo training facilitates improvements in aerobic metabolism but also improves the lactate threshold and anaerobic metabolism since the athlete sustains exercise at a higher intensity than normal. Tempo training can be done in a single 20–30-minute bout or with intervals interspersed with recovery.

Interval Training in Aerobic Conditioning

Interval training is characterized by alternating work periods and rest periods, though the intensities and durations of the work/rest periods will vary depending on the exercise objective. Athletes should not use interval training until they have built an aerobic endurance base of being able to sustain at least 20–30 minutes of steady-state exercise.

In aerobic conditioning, interval training typically uses 3–5-minute intervals with a 1:1 work to rest ratio. Interval training improves VO_2 max, lactate threshold, and anaerobic metabolism because it allows working briefly at high intensities that could not be otherwise sustained for longer periods.

High-intensity interval training (HIIT) has higher-intensity work periods (at or above 90% of VO_2 max) performed for shorter durations (30–90 seconds). A 1:1 work-to-rest ratio may be used, or recovery periods may be longer (up to 1:5) to maintain high-quality effort for each interval. Training with HIIT improves anaerobic metabolism, lactate threshold, and running speed.

Fartlek ("speed play") involves loosely structured, lower-intensity work alternated with working at higher intensities or inclines. In general, the athlete selects the paces and how often they will vary. Besides aerobic and anaerobic adaptations, Fartlek can allow the athlete to self-manage recovery and avoid overtraining.

Safety Considerations for Aerobic Endurance Training Machines

The main safety technique for the treadmill is to have the athlete straddle the belt and hold the handrails while a suitable warm-up speed is set. They can then step on while holding the handrails and using a pawing motion with one foot. Other aerobic endurance training machines like the stair stepper and elliptical trainer also have handrails that the athlete should hold onto before stepping onto the machine and starting it.

For the stationary bike, the seat height must be set accurately based on the athlete's height. The leg extended at the bottom of the pedal stroke should have a slight bend in it with the knee over the center of the pedal. The athlete should maintain a neutral spine whether pedaling upright or leaning forward.

For the rowing machine, the athlete initiates the movement with a straight back, extending the hips and knees while pulling the rower handle with the arms. The athlete finishes the rowing pull with legs fully extended, arms bent, the rowing handle just below the ribcage, and the spine straight and slightly leaning backward. The athlete will bend the knees and hips and straighten the arms to return to the starting position.

Interval Training in Anaerobic Conditioning

Interval training can be used in both aerobic and anaerobic conditioning, but its use in anaerobic conditioning must be aligned with anaerobic system energy demands to best facilitate positive adaptations. An athlete whose activities are primarily anaerobic will primarily use the phosphagen system and/or anaerobic glycolysis, though all energy systems are active at any given time.

The phosphagen system is the primary energy system during near-maximal, very short-duration activities. It requires the highest work-to-rest ratio in interval training. A 1:12 to 1:20 ratio is best, as this will facilitate adequate recovery from the near-maximal activities.

Anaerobic glycolysis is used in moderate to high-intensity activity lasting up to a few minutes. A work-to-rest ratio ranging from 1:3 to 1:5 will allow athletes to recover enough to maintain high quality and pace for each interval.

Interval training is a high-stress activity for the body and can produce overload beyond the athlete's capabilities if done too often. In general, interval training for anaerobic athletes should not be done more than 1–2 times per week.

How to Evaluate the Demands of a Sport to Influence Anaerobic Training Design

Different sports have different physiological demands, so it is important to evaluate aspects like primary energy system(s), work-to-rest ratios, and movement patterns when designing anaerobic training to improve anaerobic metabolism and adaptations. In addition, sports and activities that are primarily aerobic can benefit from some measure of anaerobic training to increase adaptations like improved speed and lactate threshold.

For example, anaerobic training for runners and sprinters will typically use running as the primary mode and involve some type of interval training at high intensities to near-maximal intensities. Anaerobic training for sports with more dynamic and unpredictable aspects, like basketball or football, will benefit from using a variety of modes and movement patterns. While high-intensity interval training involving movements like sprints would be beneficial, these athletes also need to generate large amounts of force to accelerate and change directions. Therefore, anaerobic training in these contexts could include explosive movements like Olympic lifts and plyometrics. These movements recruit fast-twitch muscle fibers and will facilitate adaptations in anaerobic energy systems when done consistently over time in training.

Tapering

Tapering is reducing training load in preparation for a competition or event so that the athlete is at peak performance on the day of competition. It is different from deloading, which is a planned phase of reducing training as a part of training cycle recovery. Tapering can be applied to both aerobic and anaerobic activities. The structure and length of the taper can depend on the nature of the event. The duration of the taper can last from 7 to 28 weeks. Typically, a longer event will warrant a longer tapering period, and a shorter event will use a shorter tapering period. For example, a marathoner may taper for a few consecutive weeks, while a sprinter may taper for a week or less. Tapering can involve reducing the duration and intensity of training while maintaining the frequency or reducing the training volume while maintaining both frequency and intensity. Typically, however, it is important to maintain the intensity during a taper so that the athlete does not experience a detraining effect and lose physiological adaptations.

Recovery Techniques

Assess an Athlete's Status to Determine Recovery Needs

There are a few simple ways to assess an athlete's status to determine recovery needs. The main objective is to prevent overtraining, as continuing to overload an athlete when recovery is needed can impair performance. First off, simple questionnaires can be used to monitor factors like stress, sleep, and energy. An athlete who reports consistently poor sleep, high stress, and low energy will need additional recovery time and considerations from workouts.

Second, resting heart rate can be used to gauge recovery. To achieve the highest level of accuracy, an athlete should measure their resting heart rate right after waking up, before getting out of bed. Doing this each day for at least a few days will provide a baseline average of a normal resting heart rate. Once a baseline average is obtained, an athlete can compare each daily measurement to the average. A resting heart rate that is higher by more than a few beats per minute can indicate that the body needs more recovery from training. Devices like heart rate monitors and smart watches also often have capabilities to assess heart rate trends and provide feedback on recovery status.

Recovery from Training

Strategies for **recovery from training** can be broadly categorized into either refueling depleted muscles or allowing muscles time to recover and repair (including the daily requirement of adequate sleep).

Nutritionally, adequate calories and macronutrients are an essential part of recovery. For example, muscle glycogen cannot be replenished without adequate carbohydrate consumption. Replenishing fluids is also vital for recovery, since dehydration can impair performance, and clients may require added electrolytes depending on the nature of their activity.

The amount of time needed for muscle recovery and repair is proportional to the amount of muscle used and the intensity. For example, a client who has participated in 1-RM attempts may need multiple recovery days versus a client who did a submaximal aerobic training bout. Longer-term excessive training (**overtraining**) may warrant multiple days to weeks for recovery. **Tapering**, a planned training volume reduction, may be used as a recovery strategy as well. **Cross-training** is a way to enhance muscle recovery while maintaining physical activity, as it uses different muscle groups than the client's given activity. For example, a runner who incorporates swimming for cross-training can maintain their fitness while reducing the amount of repetitive impact and stress on muscles and bones.

Exercise Selection to Promote Recovery

Recovery is a necessary part of training for a sport and should be intentionally incorporated into program design. While complete rest is sometimes necessary, recovery can be "active" through movements that minimize stress on the body and are restorative in nature. These movements or exercises are typically done at lighter loads, lower intensities, and/or enhance full ranges of motion. For example, a recovery or "deload" week done after a cycle of heavy resistance training might include intensities at no more than 55% of 1-RM for weighted movements along with a greater focus on bodyweight exercises. Recovery from cardiovascular training could involve lower-intensity activity and/or **cross-training** (using alternate forms of aerobic exercise to minimize stress on often-used muscle groups). Recovery through movement can also involve modes that enhance mobility and flexibility. For example, self-myofascial release, stretching, and modes like yoga can all be used to improve blood flow to muscles by moving through varied ranges of motion without imposing intense stimuli upon them.

Self-Myofascial Release

Self-myofascial release (SMR) uses tools such as foam rollers, massage sticks, or small balls to apply pressure to muscle and fascia with the objective of releasing muscle tension and facilitating more effective movement. A foam roller can be used on most major muscle groups, such as the latissimus dorsi, quadriceps, gluteals, and calves, while smaller implements (such as a tennis ball or lacrosse ball) are better to target smaller muscles, such as the pectorals, upper back, or feet.

SMR can be done before a workout to enhance range of motion or after a workout to promote recovery. When done after a workout, pairing SMR with static stretching is even more effective at increasing range of motion. A general protocol for using SMR is to spend 2 minutes slowly rolling over the length of the muscle. It is important not to move too quickly—pausing on spots that feel particularly tender or tight is more effective than quickly passing over them. In general, maintain a neutral spine when using SMR, do not roll directly over bones, do not roll acute injuries, and focus on breathing deeply and relaxing the muscles.

How to Assess Areas for Self-Myofascial Release

Self-myofascial release (SMR) is a beneficial recovery technique for athletes, but time constraints often necessitate prioritizing a few important muscle groups to target. The movement patterns of the sport or activity should be a factor in selecting SMR areas. For example, running requires repeated hip flexion and extension, as well as ankle dorsiflexion and plantar flexion, so the quadriceps, hamstrings, and calves all would be logical priority areas for SMR. Depending on the nature of the activity, movement patterns can differ from day-to-day. For example, a powerlifter would logically focus more on lower body SMR on days with squatting and deadlifting and more on upper body SMR on bench pressing days.

Specific athlete needs can also provide direction on SMR areas. Areas that are chronically tight or have restricted range of motion compared to normal ranges of motion will benefit from consistent SMR, especially when paired with static stretching. Areas of previous injury can have more adhesions in the muscle fascia as part of the healing process, so these also may be particularly useful to target with SMR for individualizing an athlete's program.

Compression Therapy

The main principle behind **compression therapy** is that having extra pressure applied to muscles improves circulation and, therefore, improves recovery. More specifically, compression therapy is intended increase blood flow to and from the muscles, carrying away waste products and boosting nutrient-rich blood. The effects of this are reduced inflammation, pain, swelling, and soreness.

Compression therapy can be used by wearing special compression garments, such as compression socks or sleeves, after a training session or competition. Specialized compression devices also exist, such as compression suits that completely cover the limbs. These work by providing dynamic air compression through a battery-powered inflating and deflating pump action. Studies on athletes who do repetitive lower body motions in their sports, such as runners and cyclists, have shown that compression therapy improves recovery after training.

Cryotherapy

Cryotherapy is a type of recovery technique where cold temperatures are used for therapeutic purposes. This can range from applying cold to localized areas, such as putting ice or a cold pack on an injury, to whole-body cryotherapy where an athlete is immersed in an ice bath or a specialized cold chamber for a few minutes.

One of the main reasons for using cryotherapy as a recovery technique is for its quality of transient **vasoconstriction**, or causing blood vessels to temporarily narrow. Vasoconstriction can reduce muscle soreness and decrease the body's inflammatory response, promoting quicker recovery after exercise. The vasoconstriction associated with cryotherapy also decreases the body's core temperature, which can be especially useful for recovery after training at very intense levels or in a hot environment. There is also evidence showing that whole-body cryotherapy can benefit sleep through alleviating pain and activating the parasympathetic nervous system, which promotes a relaxation response.

Heat Therapy

Similar to cryotherapy, heat therapy can be used in localized areas, such as a heating pack on a sore muscle, or as a full-body recovery modality, such as immersion in a hot tub, sauna, or steam room. Heat therapy causes **vasodilation,** which is the widening of blood vessels. This allows more blood to flow through the vessels. This accelerates the flow of nutrients to muscle tissue as well as the removal of waste products. Heat therapy can also have a beneficial effect on connective tissue by improving range of motion and elasticity; however, heat therapy is contraindicated for acute injuries because the vasodilation can increase swelling and inflammation in the injured area. In addition, heat therapy should be used with caution when skin is coming into direct contact with heat sources, as they can cause burns.

Contrast Hydrotherapy

Contrast hydrotherapy consists of immersing a limb or the entire body in water while alternating periods of hot and cold temperatures. Temperature changes occur every 30 seconds to 3 minutes for a total of 10–15 minutes. The premise behind contrast hydrotherapy is that alternating between vasoconstriction (provoked by cold) and vasodilation (provoked by heat) enhances circulation beyond using just heat or cold as a single modality. Contrast hydrotherapy is most typically used in post-exercise recovery to reduce pain, swelling, and inflammation.

There is less evidence for contrast therapy's effectiveness than using heat or cold therapies by themselves, though reported benefits of contrast hydrotherapy include reduced fatigue and muscle soreness after training. The cold temperatures in cryotherapy can be uncomfortable, so contrast therapy can provide a more bearable way to undergo cold therapy because the cold is interspersed with periods of rewarming.

Program Implementation

Motor Learning and Skill Acquisition Techniques

Feedback

It is important to provide specific and constructive feedback so that individuals can understand how to improve and correct errors and receive motivation and reinforcement on what they are doing well. There are two main types of feedback. **Intrinsic feedback** comes from within the individual by their own senses, such as what they felt after missing a lift. **Augmented feedback** comes from outside of the individual by an external source, such as a video or a coach showing the athlete where a technique error was made. When an individual receives augmented feedback, this can provide one of two types of information to enhance learning outcomes. **Knowledge of results** involves information on the outcome of a movement or task in relation to its goal (e.g., the recorded split times for running intervals or the percentage of free throw shots made). **Knowledge of performance** involves information about movement patterns—for example, what a coach notices about an athlete's gait or technique that may need slight changes to be more effective.

Whole Practice and Part Practice

Practicing a skill can be structured into whole practice or part practice. In **whole practice**, the skill is learned as one complete unit rather than it being broken down into parts. Whole practice is best used when a skill is not complex and when the parts of the skill are highly interrelated. An example of this would be a sprint, where it would not necessarily be logical to separate the arm drive from the leg turnover involved. In **part practice**, the skill is learned in phases with the eventual aim of combining the phases back into performing the skill smoothly. Part practice is most suitable when the task is more complex and has phases with logical transition points from one to the next that can be isolated. For example, the Olympic lifts involve a first, second, and third pull, and the technique of each could be practiced individually before combining them together.

Methods of Part Practice

Part practice involves breaking a skill down into phases. There are three main types. **Simplification** reduces the movement challenge by lowering the intensity, such as through slower speed or lighter weight (e.g., a slow tempo back squat with an empty bar). **Segmentation** splits a more complex skill into individual phases, such as breaking down the Olympic lifts into each individual pull. **Fractionalization** takes components that normally occur simultaneously and provides independent component practice, like a basketball layup with independent practice on shooting and dribbling.

Integrating parts back into the whole can be done in three ways. In **pure-part training**, phases are returned into the whole movement once each phase has been successfully practiced on its own multiple times. In **progressive-part training**, phases are practiced in isolation. Each successive phase is done by itself before adding it on to a series of multiple phases. In **repetitive-part training**, phases are practiced in a stepwise manner by adding phases one by one until the skill is integrated. For example, a skill with five parts might involve practicing parts one and two, then adding the third part to do the first three parts in a row, and so on.

Types of Practice Schedules

Blocked practice is a typical way to learn skills where individuals do the same skill multiple times before proceeding to the next skill. For example, a team that has three skills to practice would complete all their practice on the first skill before moving to the second skill, and so on. **Random practice** puts planned skills in an unstructured order. For example, a team with the same three skills to practice would rotate among the skills, mixing up the skill order rather than having them in a set structure. **Variable practice** uses a variety of movements and fluctuations in practice conditions rather than focusing on single specific skills. For example, football athletes practicing agility in defense might use various distances and pieces of equipment rather than doing the same drill repeatedly. Integrating each type of practice is optimal for motor skill learning. Blocked practice results in more skilled performance during the practice session itself, while random practice and variable practice facilitate learning by promoting cognitive flexibility with unfamiliar or changing conditions.

Feedback and Motor Skill Learning Stages

The Fitts and Posner model of motor learning proposes that there are three skill levels through which an individual progresses. In the **cognitive stage**, the movements are new. They must think through the details of how to do the movements in order to avoid mistakes. Feedback in the cognitive stage should focus on building confidence with the fundamentals of the movement, avoiding small details that might become overwhelming. In the **associative stage**, the individual grasps the basic idea of the movement from building skill and efficiency in doing it but still needs to focus to avoid errors. Feedback to individuals in the associative stage can focus on details and urge them to focus only on relevant cues. In the **autonomous stage**, the individual has done the movement many times, and the repetitive practice has honed efficient, skilled movements that do not require effortful conscious thought. Feedback for individuals in the autonomous stage may focus on minor corrections and keeping the mind calm rather than fixating excessively on movement details or distracting thoughts.

Instructional Strategies

There are three main types of instructional styles that can be conceptualized on a continuum from most detailed to least detailed, and each type of instruction has use depending on the context and athlete. **Explicit instructions** are the most detailed and outline all main aspects of the movement or task. For example, explicit instructions for an Olympic lift would detail what happens during each pull and the proper body position during each pull. **Guided discovery** provides key instructions without explicit details, enabling some cognitive exploration from the individual on how to do the task most efficiently. In the Olympic lift example, the individual might get a reminder on receiving the bar in a squat with a straight spine but will not receive more specific details on how to execute the end of the lift. **Discovery** provides minimal to no direction, only the main goal to accomplish. Using the Olympic lift example, the athlete might simply be told to get the bar from the ground to overhead, allowing them to explore ways this could be done.

Internal and External Cueing

A **cue** is instruction provided to enhance performance. **Internal cues** emphasize focusing attention within oneself. Such cues could include how to move a body segment or what to feel within a muscle group during a movement—for example, giving cues to bend at the knees or to brace the abdominals. **External cues** emphasize focusing attention on aspects outside of oneself. These external aspects could include the environment, the equipment, teammates, opponents, etc. Examples of external cues could include instructing an individual where to land on the floor with a jumping movement or to watch for a teammate as they dribble a basketball. Cues can be **auditory** (verbal instruction), **visual** (observation and demonstration), and **kinesthetic** (guidance on what to feel or hands-on corrections). There are individual differences in comprehending cues, so the nature and number of cues should be adapted to each personal preference.

Evidence-Based Tests to Maximize Test Reliability and Validity

Benefits of Testing

Testing benefits athletes and coaches in four ways. First, testing can be used in goal setting. Providing baseline measurements at the start of a season, paired with a properly periodized plan and coaching, can help motivate athletes to improve on the test when it is performed again. Related to goal setting, tests can be used to evaluate progress over the course of the season or another given time period. For example, if an athlete sets a goal to improve their 1-RM back squat by 10% over 6 months, it would be logical to test their 1-RM at the halfway point to gauge their progress or whether the goal needs to be reevaluated.

Testing can also be used to identify athletic talent. This is especially important for athletes who are new to the techniques and rules of the sport. While an individual's sport-specific knowledge might be minimal, testing could reveal significant talent in aspects like strength and speed, highlighting their high potential to eventually excel in the sport. Identifying areas for improvement is another important function of tests. Most sports have multiple relevant components (such as speed, strength, power, etc.), so doing multiple types of tests can highlight where an athlete may need additional focused training.

Test Selection

Primary Considerations

Two main areas in test selection are sports specificity and individualization. Under the realm of sport specificity, a test should use the same or similar biomechanical movement patterns as the sport. For example, an agility test would have direct application to a sport with frequent and consistent changes of direction like football or basketball. Another aspect of sport specificity is to consider the primary metabolic energy system used in the sport. For example, baseball involves short, near-maximal bursts of energy with throwing and running, so anaerobic tests would be more relevant than aerobic tests.

Individualization, or considering the right type of test for each individual, should first take training status and experience into account. For example, a group of adolescent football athletes who are new to the sport do not have the experience to be tested on the power clean, which requires high levels of technical expertise. Individualization should also account for age and sex. Younger athletes may need developmentally appropriate tests that are easy to instruct and demonstrate and do not require intensive technique. Differences in female athletes, such as body composition and muscular strength, mean that some tests will be less valid than others.

Sport

Fitness testing can significantly differ across various sports based on unique physical and physiological demands. For example, basketball and volleyball require quick movements, sprinting, and jumping. Tests for agility, speed, vertical jump, and upper body power are all relevant for activities like moving quickly on the court, blocking defenders or serves, and jumping for a layup or a spike. Long-distance sports like running and cycling require sustained aerobic energy production. VO_2 max testing, or testing aerobic capacity through field tests, would be one of the most relevant tests to assess fitness level and gauge progress. Contact sports like boxing and wrestling would benefit from tests measuring aspects like anaerobic capacity and upper body power. Anaerobic capacity is needed to maintain high-intensity effort during rounds, and upper body power is needed for striking and grappling. A sport like gymnastics requires high levels of full-body flexibility and balance, so these types of tests would be a high priority, along with tests for upper and lower body strength and power that are relevant for skills like tumbling and vaulting. Overall, sport-specific testing facilitates the development of tailored training programs to further enhance sport skills.

Sport Positions

For many types of sports, different positions require different physical and physiological attributes. This can make testing selection significantly varied across all individuals on the team. For example, football wide receivers need to have high levels of speed and agility for their position, while linemen need high levels of strength and power to withstand and apply force. As another example, in soccer, a goalkeeper's most relevant tests might include ones for agility, reaction time, and explosive power, while a midfielder's most relevant tests might include ones for agility, speed, and aerobic endurance. Position-specific fitness testing will be more accurate in assessing athletes' readiness and abilities for their roles than using a general approach for all athletes. Using a position-specific approach in testing can then guide the structure of individualizing training programs, enhancing overall team performance.

Considerations for Athlete Health

Before starting any physical activity, including testing, it is crucial to conduct a preparticipation screening and obtain medical clearance. This ensures the athlete's safety by identifying any health conditions or physical aspects that may exclude an athlete from participating, warrant contraindications, or require specific accommodation. As an example of a contraindication, 1-RM tests are typically not recommended for individuals with high blood pressure due to the additional strain that lifting maximal loads places on the heart. In this case, a safer alternative would be estimating the 1-RM from a submaximal test with multiple repetitions. As an example of specific accommodation, an athlete with asthma might be cleared to participate with the stipulation that they need extra time to warm up and must have their inhaler within reach during cardiovascular testing.

It is also important to consider the athlete's psychological or mental health. High stress or anxiety levels can negatively affect performance, so it might be best to postpone a test if an athlete is facing significant challenges. Additionally, certain tests might be psychologically distressing for some athletes and should be avoided. For example, measuring weight or body composition could be triggering for an individual with a history of disordered eating.

Equipment Use and Calibration

Proper equipment use and calibration ensures accurate and reliable results. All personnel administering tests should be familiar with the equipment and have used it multiple times. Some equipment can be complex and require specific knowledge, like the technology used for force plates or underwater weighing to assess body composition. Improper equipment use can lead to inaccurate test measurements or even increased risk of athlete injury.

Equipment can also have unique calibration procedures required for accuracy. For example, skinfold calipers, used for measuring body composition, should be calibrated regularly to ensure they are accurate. Otherwise, a false reading could give an inaccurate assessment of an athlete's body composition. Similarly, a force plate used for a static vertical jump should be regularly checked for correct function and accuracy. Inaccuracies could lead to an overestimation or underestimation of an athlete's muscular power. This could misinform the training program, leading to ineffective training or increased injury risk.

The Role of Trained Personnel

Personnel administering tests should be well-trained in safety, accuracy, and consistency. It is helpful for a well-trained individual, such as the strength and conditioning professional, to act as the test supervisor if there are multiple tests going on at once or large groups with multiple testers. Well before the actual testing takes place (such as in the days or weeks prior), the testing supervisor should plan and practice the test format ahead of time with staff, going through aspects like how to record results or how to operate equipment. Having consistent protocols across all testers is another critical aspect for efficiency and accuracy. For example, if one tester provides a 5-minute warm-up and another tester provides a 15-minute warm-up, the results may be affected, and one group will take longer, detracting from efficiency. Also, having enough personnel can help manage large groups of athletes and minimize wait time. For example, a group doing four different local muscular endurance tests can be split into four groups and rotate among testers, with each tester responsible for one specific test.

Scheduling

First, tests should be scheduled in a logical order, considering factors like fatigue and the influence of tests on each other. For example, a non-fatiguing test like body composition should be done before a maximal power test because body composition measurements will not detract from physical performance. Scheduling adequate rest between tests is important, particularly if they target similar muscle groups or energy systems. For example, doing both a 1-RM back squat and a 40-m sprint test will require rest not only for anaerobic energy system recovery but to avoid excessive fatigue of the leg muscles as well.

Scheduling should also consider optimal times of day for testing, if applicable. For example, tests like body composition are often most accurate if they are done in a fasted state, so early morning would be a preferable time for these. Optimal times for athletes are also a consideration. While not every athlete's time preferences can necessarily be accommodated, some athletes may perform better in the morning, and others may prefer the afternoon, for instance.

Testing and Monitoring Protocols and Procedures

Enhancing Athlete Readiness for Testing

Enhancing athlete readiness for testing has both mental and physical aspects. Mental preparation for testing centers around giving athletes clear instruction in advance, such as days before the test, so that they know what to expect and can ask questions. It is also typically valuable to provide lower-intensity practice tests 1–3 days before testing as a way of 'rehearsing' how the test will go.

Knowing about testing details well ahead of time also allows athletes to account for any behaviors or factors that could affect the accuracy of test results. For example, an athlete should avoid intense workouts in the days leading up to an intense test, like a 1-RM or a maximum muscular power test. Enhancing physical readiness on the testing day itself is done through an appropriate warm-up. While different tests require different types of warm-ups, the overall structure is a general warm-up (such as moderate intensity aerobic activity and dynamic movements for all major joints through full ranges of motion) followed by a specific warm-up that more closely mimics movements in the test.

Conducting Multiple Tests

A fundamental aspect of conducting multiple tests is ensuring that tests do not interfere with each other in respect to athlete performance. For example, tests for anaerobic and aerobic capacity are both fatiguing and require longer amounts of recovery time. It would affect the accuracy of the second test if these were done in the same day with minimal rest between. While dedicating a day to testing and performing a battery of tests can be time efficient, spreading tests out over multiple days can improve test accuracy.

If doing multiple tests, non-fatiguing tests should go first since they will not affect the next tests performed. Non-fatiguing tests include body composition, anthropometric measures, and flexibility. The next three types of tests in order are agility tests, tests for maximal power and strength (like 1-RM), and sprint tests. These types of tests are more technical and require brief, high-intensity efforts, making them a higher priority in the testing order. The next three types of tests in order are muscular endurance tests, anaerobic capacity tests, and aerobic capacity tests. If adequate recovery is provided, these are not likely to be affected by any previously performed tests.

Testing for Maximum Muscular Strength

Maximum muscular strength is commonly assessed through 1-repetition maximum (1-RM) testing. Lifts chosen for 1-RM are typically multi-joint movements for large muscle groups, such as the bench press, shoulder press, squat, and deadlift. For safety, athletes should never be assessed on lifts in which they have minimal to no experience. At least one spotter is typically needed, depending on the lift. If there is a chance of the athlete dropping the bar in failing the lift (such as failing to rise out of the bottom of a back squat), the athlete should either lift in a rack with safety pins or lift with bumper plates in an area where the bar can be safely dropped on the floor.

The testing area should have a variety of weight plates that allow gradual increases in resistance up to the athlete's 1-RM. The athlete starts with 5–10 repetitions at a light resistance, rests 1 minute, does 3–5 repetitions at a moderate resistance, rests 2 minutes, then continues increasing resistance, typically in even increments, with 2–4 minutes between attempts until a 1-RM is reached. Obtaining the 1-RM in 3–5 testing sets is ideal to minimize unnecessary fatigue.

Testing for Maximum Muscular Power

Maximum muscular power can be tested in a variety of ways. Power exercises, such as the Olympic lifts and their variations, can be tested via 1-RM. The same general protocols apply across all 1-RM lifts, such as gradual increases, resting 2–4 minutes between attempts, and attempting to obtain the 1-RM in 3–5 testing sets. The primary difference with 1-RM testing for Olympic lifts is that they are not spotted, and the athlete should have an environment and equipment that permits safely dropping the bar if they need to bail from the lift.

Other movements can be used for testing maximum muscular power, such as the standing long jump, types of vertical jump, **reactive strength index** using a mat that measures contact time, and the **Margaria-Kalamen test**, which involves sprinting up a 9-step staircase 3 steps at a time as fast as possible from a 20 foot (6 meter) standing start. General protocols for all these tests include providing time for lower-intensity practice trials as part of the warm-up, using the best of three trials in the testing results, and providing 2–3 minutes of recovery between trials.

Testing for Anaerobic and Aerobic Capacity

Like other fatiguing tests, athletes should go through a warm-up and have lower-intensity practice trials to anticipate what to expect in anaerobic or aerobic testing. A common test for anaerobic capacity is the **300-yard shuttle**, which requires an open area like a field with enough room for a 25-yard sprint. The athlete sprints from the starting line to the 25-yard line and back, then completes the sprint five more times for a total of six down-and-back sprints. Multiple athletes can be tested at once as long as there is a line judge for each athlete. A second trial is done after a 5-minute rest period, and the average of both trials is recorded as the score.

Common tests for aerobic capacity involve either the athlete running as fast as they can for a preset distance (such as the **1.5-mile run**) or the athlete covering as much distance as they can within a preset time (such as the **12-minute run**). These tests require a measured course or a track. The **Yo-Yo intermittent recovery test** and the **maximal aerobic speed test** are two other tests for aerobic capacity, both of which involve maintaining gradually increasing speed until failure.

Testing for Local Muscular Endurance

General protocols for tests of local muscular endurance involve either accumulating as many repetitions of a movement as possible or lifting a submaximal load repeatedly until failure. Like many other types of tests, it is vital to not only provide a warm-up but to provide instruction on correct repetitions so that the test is accurate. Most bodyweight resistance training movements, such as partial curl-ups, push-ups, squats, and pull-ups, lend themselves well to local muscular endurance testing. Some test protocols involve performing the movement in time with a metronome. An example of this is the **partial curl-up test**, where the athlete curls up in time with 40 beats per minute until failure or reaching 75 curl-ups. Other test protocols involve submaximal external resistance, such as the **YMCA bench press test** with a load of 80 lb (36 kg) for males and 35 lb (16 kg) for females. In this test, the load is lifted and lowered in time with a metronome cadence of 60 beats per minute. Some local muscular endurance tests have standards that vary based on athlete sex—for example, in the **push-up test**, females perform the movement with knees on the ground, while males use a straight body position.

Testing for Speed and Agility

The most typical tests for speed are straight line sprints that evaluate speed over a set distance, such as 10 meters or 40 yards (37 meters). The testing distance should be chosen based on relevance to the sport. For example, 10 meters is not long enough to reach top speed and is better suited for sports with brief bursts of acceleration.

Many agility tests use predetermined changes of direction or multidirectional running. The **pro agility test** (also known as the 20-yard shuttle) and the **505 agility test** both assess change of direction speed with sprinting to points on a measured course and using the best score of two trials. The **T-test** assesses athletes by having them sprint forward in a straight line, shuffling laterally, and run backwards in a T-shaped pattern on a measured course. It uses the best score of two trials. The **hexagon test** is unique from the previously described agility tests, as it involves changes of direction with double-leg hopping in and out of a measured hexagon shape rather than running.

Dynamic stretching is important to include in pre-test warm-ups since these tests often involve maximal effort. Going through full ranges of motion with test-specific and sport-specific movements can help prevent injury.

Testing for Balance and Stability

Two main tests for balance and stability are the **balance error scoring system (BESS)** and the **star excursion balance test (SEBT).** The BESS assesses static postural stability over three different body positions on two different surfaces—a firm surface, like the floor, and a soft surface with some instability, like a foam pad. The body positions include standing on both legs with the feet together, balancing on the non-dominant foot with the other leg flexed to 90°, and assuming a tandem stance with the dominant foot in front. Each position is tested for up to 20 seconds with the eyes closed and the hands on the hips. The sum of the scores makes up the test result.

The SEBT assesses single-leg stability in various directions. It is done on a grid with 8 lines evenly spaced every 45°, which can be created using tape on the floor. The athlete stands in the center of the grid on one leg and reaches as far as they can on each of the 8 lines, returning to the center after each reach. The athlete's score is based off the average of 3 trials for each leg. For both tests, errors like losing balance or moving out of body position end the trial.

Testing for Flexibility

While flexibility tests are considered non-fatiguing tests, they require a thorough warm-up that includes dynamic and static stretches to prevent injuries such as muscle strains. A common flexibility test is the **sit-and-reach test**, which can be done with a measuring tape on the floor or with a sit-and-reach box. The athlete sits shoeless with their legs extended and feet 12 inches apart and reaches forward as far as they can on the tape or the box, exhaling during the greatest part of the stretch and keeping their hands lined up evenly over each other. Three trials with approximately 1 minute of rest between each are performed, with the best trial scored.

The **overhead squat** test is a dynamic movement rather than a static stretch and assesses the athlete's full-body stability and mobility. The athlete performs a squat below parallel with arms extended overhead holding a dowel or barbell, repeating the squat at least five times so that their movement patterns can be observed. Scoring this test is not numerical but based on gauging if the athlete can successfully overhead squat with minimal to no errors. Errors include arms falling forward, heels lifting, torso leaning forward, and not maintaining a neutral spine.

Anthropometric Measurements

Anthropometric measurements are ones that provide objective data about body size, such as weight, height, and circumferences (e.g., waist measurement). Weight should be measured with a regularly calibrated scale, such as a balance scale or an electronic scale. If possible, for most accuracy, athletes should be measured in a fasted state, like early in the morning. Sweating can create weight fluctuations as body water is lost, so it is best to weigh athletes before they have exercised and while wearing dry, lightweight clothing. Height should be measured with the athlete standing in socks or barefoot against a flat wall and using a stadiometer, which has a sliding part adjustable with the top of the head, or with a measuring tape.

Body circumferences, also known as body girths, are measured with a tape measure. These measurements may be used to assess if an athlete has increased in muscle mass or if an athlete has lost body fat. Various common measurement sites include the abdomen, quadriceps, and biceps. The tape should be snug and level over the body segment, and the athlete should stand with normal posture, neither flexing the muscle nor trying to contract it (such as sucking the stomach in).

Skinfold Measurements

Skinfold Calipers

Skinfold calipers are spring-loaded instruments that provide an estimate of body composition through measuring subcutaneous fat. Depending on the equation used, a range of three to eight different skinfold sites are used to estimate body composition. The sites can be invasive in requiring athletes to reveal sites often covered by clothing, such as the chest skinfold or the suprailiac skinfold, so a private space for testing is important.

Each site has specific anatomical landmarks for accuracy and should be marked with a pen or marker before taking a skinfold. The tester will grasp the site firmly with their thumb and fingers to make a skinfold, possibly needing to roll or 'knead' the skin slightly to pull it away from the muscle. The prongs of the caliper should be placed perpendicular to the fold in its center (or approximately 0.5–1 inch (1–2 cm) away from the thumb and fingers holding it). Next, the tester should release the caliper grip while still holding the skinfold. Allowing 1–2 seconds for the caliper to sink into the skin provides a more accurate reading. At least two measurements are taken at each site, with additional measurements potentially needed to achieve the highest level of accuracy.

Sites for Skinfold Measurements

There are eight different commonly used sites. The chest skinfold is diagonal, halfway between the anterior axillary line and the nipple. The midaxillary skinfold is vertical, in line with the sternum's xiphoid process on the midaxillary line. The triceps skinfold is vertical, halfway between the shoulder joint and elbow joint. The subscapular skinfold is diagonal, on a line from the vertebral border to 0.5–1 inch from the scapula's inferior angle. The abdominal skinfold is vertical, 1 inch to the right of the navel. The suprailiac skinfold is diagonal, above the ilium and aligned with a descending line from the anterior axilla. The thigh skinfold is vertical and anterior on the thigh, halfway between the hip joint and the center of the patella. The calf skinfold is vertical and medial on the calf, taken at maximal calf circumference.

Different skinfold equations exist, and some do not use all eight sites. For example, a common three-site equation uses the chest, abdomen, and thigh skinfold for males, and the triceps, suprailium, and thigh skinfold for females.

Evaluate and Interpret Results

Improving Validity

The **validity** of a test is its ability to accurately measure what it is designed to measure. A main factor in valid results is having standardized procedures for testing and keeping them consistent across all athletes. For example, a 1-RM test administered to multiple football athletes should be done in the same environment and with the same equipment, same warm-up and rest periods, and same instructions provided to the athletes before and during the test. Another factor is ensuring that the test is specific to the sport. For example, an aerobic capacity test like the 1.5-mile run would be less valid for basketball athletes than a test on anaerobic capacity and/or agility since the sport involves short, higher-intensity bursts of activity. Ensuring that tests are appropriate for an athlete's skill level also enhances validity. A 1-RM test may be less valid at assessing maximal strength in a novice who lacks experience with the lift. Valid tests also are objective, with some type of numerical analysis that connects test results and performance. For example, measurements on the vertical jump test for a volleyball player would correlate well with the ability to block a spike over the net from the other team.

High and Low Validity

Test situations that support high validity include objective results, sports specificity, and relevance to the athlete. For example, valid test situations for a sprinter could include using the standing long jump or the Margaria-Kalamen test, since both assess explosive lower body power, which is directly relevant for sprinting. Testing a 1-RM power clean would also be valid for muscular power as long as the athlete is experienced with the movement.

A primary error in testing validity is choosing a test that is not as directly relevant or applicable to the sport. For example, if a long-distance runner is tested on local muscular endurance through the YMCA bench press test, this test will have lower validity for their performance. While muscular endurance is important in the sport, lower body endurance is a much higher determinant of performance than upper body endurance. As another example, if swim team athletes are tested on aerobic capacity and the 12-minute run test is performed, the results will lack validity because the aerobic demands of running are different from those of swimming. In this case, research would need to be done for selecting a valid swimming test for aerobic capacity.

CONSIDERATIONS FOR TEST VALIDITY IN TESTING STRENGTH AND POWER

Both muscular strength and muscular power are measures of a muscle's ability to exert force; however, it is important to differentiate between low- and high-speed strength and power when choosing a valid test for an athlete's sport and situation. **Low-speed muscular strength** is most accurately tested through 1-RM lifts or isometric strength measurements. Some sports require the ability to contract muscles rapidly and exert high levels of force, which is **high-speed muscular strength** (also termed **maximal anaerobic muscular power** or **anaerobic power)**. Athletes requiring this quality include sprinters, high jumpers/long jumpers, and Olympic weightlifters. Valid tests for high-speed strength include 1-RMs of Olympic lifts (snatch, clean and jerk) or their variations (such as push press or hang clean), long jump or vertical jump, and the Margaria-Kalamen test.

No single test is typically the best for a given sport, and many types of sports require both low-speed and high-speed muscular strength, necessitating a battery of tests. For example, basketball and football players need low-speed strength of the lower body but also high-speed strength for jumping and blocking. Testing anaerobic power through a Wingate test with an ergometer is another option for athletes who sprint using equipment, such as a cyclist or a rowing athlete.

BIOMECHANICS AND TEST RESULTS

Biomechanics refers to the relationship between components of the musculoskeletal system (like bones, muscles, and joints) in creating movement. Individual differences in these body components can result in varied test results, even among two individuals who appear similar and play the same sport. One example is joint structure. Hip joint depth varies across human anatomy. Deeper hip sockets can limit squat depth, which might impact performance in tests for strength, power, and flexibility. Limb length is another example. An individual with longer limbs is likely to have an advantage over someone with shorter limbs in tests that involve sprinting or jumping, even if the two individuals are the same height; however, shorter limbs can be an advantage in tests for strength and power because the distance to move the weight from the ground to the ending point is reduced.

GENETICS AND TEST RESULTS

Muscle fiber composition is one genetic factor influencing test results. All humans have a combination of type I (slow-twitch) and type II (fast-twitch) fibers. While there can be small shifts in fiber type with training, genetics is a main determinant of an individual's muscle fiber make-up, which can then influence test results. For example, an individual with a higher proportion of type II fibers would typically perform better on tests involving high power and fast conduction velocities, like a 1-RM of an Olympic lift, sprint test, or jump test. Those with more type I fibers tend to perform better on tests for aerobic capacity or local muscular endurance since their muscles are more fatigue-resistant at submaximal intensities.

Hormones are another aspect that has genetic variation across individuals. Besides the hormonal differences between males and females, two individuals of the same biological sex can have different hormone levels, apart from hormonal responses to training. For example, a male with higher testosterone levels compared to another male will have greater capacity to build strength and mass and would do better on tests for strength and power.

ATHLETIC PROFILE

Evaluating performance can be done in a scientific, systematic manner through the steps of an **athletic profile**, which is a group of tests specific to a given sport's needs. First, a needs assessment is done for consideration of the most important components of the sport or activity, such as metabolic system(s), muscle groups and actions, and skills. Then, valid and reliable tests are selected that measure these components. Most sports or activities will have multiple relevant tests, and consecutive tests should be separated by appropriate recovery periods for best reliability. After administering the tests, the data can be compared with normative data and with other data from the same athlete (i.e., if tests are done at the beginning and the end of a training cycle). Test results should be applied to improve performance, such as making changes in the training cycle or individualizing components of training for athletes.

Modifying the Training Program Based on Test Results

General Considerations

Test results for an athlete can be compared to typical norms for the sport and demographic, to other athletes on the same team, or to the athlete over time (such as comparing an athlete's test results at the start and finish of the season). All three comparisons might be made, though not all sports and demographics have typical norms in the literature. Regardless of the comparison used, the results can help identify any deficits or weaknesses in the athlete and guide modifications of the program going forward. For example, an athlete who scores high on aerobic capacity but has low scores in balance and flexibility may need additional unilateral training and stretching incorporated into their program. In contrast, an athlete whose testing results show high levels of muscular strength but lower levels of agility may need their program modified to have a greater focus on multidirectional movement. Comparison of results can be especially important when multiple tests are done. This helps prioritize the greatest needs for improvement without trying to make too many programming changes at once.

Body Composition

Body composition can be one measure of health, but it is important to note that it is not the sole measure that determines performance levels. Some sports favor athletes with a low percentage of body fat (such as gymnastics, long-distance running, and rowing) or have requirements for weight class standards (such as wrestling or Olympic lifting). Guidelines for essential body fat (the body fat required for basic physiological functions) are 3% for males and 12% for females. Lower body fat than this can decrease performance and increase the risk for health issues. Most athletes compete with body fat percentages well above essential body fat; however, higher body fat percentages can also impact performance and put athletes at risk for obesity-related diseases like high cholesterol or high blood pressure.

Therefore, results of body composition testing should be interpreted considering the athlete, their sport, and implications for health and performance. Athletes with higher body fat than typical ranges may need additional nutrition guidance in their programs provided by a qualified nutrition professional. Athletes with lower body fat than typical ranges may also benefit from nutrition guidance. Athletes who weigh less than similar athletes may need adjustments to their resistance training programs to enhance lean muscle mass.

Organization and Administration

Organizational Environment

Reporting and Documentation

Effective reporting and documentation serve multiple purposes in safe facility operation. One is to establish and maintain the standards of the facility through documentation. This includes the credentials of staff and written policies and procedures. A second important purpose is to reduce injury risk. Having participants complete pre-participation documents like waivers, informed consent, and medical clearance provides a written record of their personal information and understanding of any legal risks. Other types of documentation that prevent injury risk are regular maintenance check reports and user information provided by the manufacturer. For example, verifying through regular reporting that facility treadmills are regularly checked and maintained in accordance with manufacturer instructions provides assurance that their use is less likely to cause injury. A third purpose is to establish effective emergency response. A written emergency plan and using incident reports are both documentation examples under this realm. The emergency plan facilitates efficient and effective response in case of injury (with information such as location of the AED, nearest hospital, etc.). Incident reports objectively document any injuries or accidents occurring within the facility, which allows for accurate review of circumstances and future implementation of preventive measures.

Policies and Procedures

Policies and procedures go together in facility operation in providing a framework for consistent, safe practices. **Policies** are rules that reflect program goals and objectives. For example, since safety should be a main objective of a strength and conditioning facility, a corresponding policy would be that anyone under 18 years old cannot train without staff supervision. **Procedures** provide specifics on how the policies are executed. For example, a corresponding procedure with the previous policy would be that there must be at least one strength and conditioning professional for every eight athletes under 18 years old.

Equipment use policies and procedures are another example, such as stating how equipment should be used, stored, and maintained. A policy could state that free weights should always be returned to the rack after use to minimize tripping hazards, with the corresponding procedure that staff is regularly circulating on the fitness floor to enforce this rule. As another example, a facility might have a policy that all users should wipe down their equipment after use to keep it clean and hygienic. The facility procedure could outline where wipes are located in stations throughout the fitness floor and how often they are checked and refilled.

Program Objectives

All strength and conditioning programs have program goals, though these depend on the nature of the program and participants. Goals cannot be achieved without setting specific **program objectives**, which outline how goals will be reached. For example, a general goal applicable to all strength and conditioning programs is to improve performance while preventing injuries in participants. Program objectives that align with this goal could include developing periodized programs that prevent overtraining and overuse injuries and providing comprehensive monitoring and education to participants on related aspects of health, such as nutrition.

Staffing the performance team should be aligned with being able to meet the program objectives. A collaborative team of professionals with different specialties helps this happen effectively. For example, even though a strength and conditioning professional has knowledge of injury prevention and response, a team member like an athletic trainer or physical therapist is even more well-equipped to treat and respond to injuries. Therefore, having this type of professional on staff is more effective in meeting program objectives. As another example, specialized nutrition education is best provided by a nutrition professional, so having one on staff for this primary role would also help meet program objectives.

Staff Preparedness

Staff must be prepared for the responsibilities of the role, including meeting professional standards and performing program-specific duties. This includes keeping professional certifications up to date, maintaining and enhancing knowledge on instruction methods (such as through continuing education), and understanding adherence to the program philosophy. Another critical area is emergency preparedness. This is accomplished through maintaining appropriate emergency response certification (such as CPR, AED, and first aid) and staying current on the procedures for emergency response in the facility (such as through doing emergency drills or debriefing after an emergency incident). A third area falls under the realm of program-specific, facility-specific, and governing body-specific policies, procedures, rules, and regulations. As some examples, this includes understanding legal issues and being prepared to prevent them (such as maintaining liability insurance), being proactive to prevent participant safety concerns (such as mandating preparticipation screenings), and understanding responsibilities for maintenance and cleaning within the facility.

Emergency Action Plans

An **emergency action plan** specifies in writing how emergencies should be handled. Any staff member working in the facility should be familiar with the emergency action plan, have access to it, and maintain emergency response certification (CPR, AED, and first aid). The emergency action plan should detail aspects like communication with advanced care personnel (such as the location of phones in the facility and the phone numbers for the nearest hospital, team physician, etc.). The written plan should also communicate location details that would be critical in an emergency, such as where first aid kids, AEDs, and exits are located and where an ambulance can access the facility. Emergency planning is also not limited to medical emergencies or acute injuries; the written plan should also communicate what to do in extreme weather, fire, an active shooter, and other emergencies. In an emergency, collaboration among staff allows prioritizing safety. For example, the first staff member to encounter an injured athlete might start providing care while they call for help and direct a second staff member to contact EMS, and a third staff member might be directed to secure the area to prevent interference from the public or media.

The Strength and Conditioning Facility

Phases of New Facility Design

In the **predesign phase**, the requirements of the facility are identified through a **needs analysis**, which could include the types of activities that will take place in the facility, the expected number of people using the facility, and any specific needs of the activities or individuals. For example, if the facility plans to have aquatic activities, it will need to have corresponding plumbing, ventilation, and changing rooms. A **feasibility study** then follows by evaluating strengths, weaknesses, opportunities, and threats (also known as a **SWOT analysis**) to gauge the extent of the facility's potential success. A **master plan** is drawn in the predesign phase, which includes not only the physical layout and design of the facility but also budget, staff operations, and goals. The final part of the predesign phase is hiring an architect.

In the **design phase**, a collaborative effort takes place by the design committee. The committee is typically made of professionals that will work in the facility (such as strength and conditioning professionals, athletic trainers, coaches, etc.) in partnership with the architect and local city planning personnel. Having multiple perspectives ensures that the facility will be functional and safe for use with efficient flow of traffic.

The **construction phase** is typically the longest phase, lasting from the start of facility construction until the facility is structurally complete. This phase will use and reference the master plan created in the predesign phase throughout facility construction to ensure that goals and deadlines are met. The fourth and final phase is the **preoperation phase**. Here, the facility is completely built but is not yet fully functional, as it requires furnishings and staff. Decisions for hiring staff should align with facility requirements and activity qualifications. For example, if public aquatic activities are offered, lifeguards will need to be part of the staffing, or if competitive sports activities will take place on-site, athletic trainers should be hired. Additionally, aspects of daily facility function should be determined before the facility opens. For example, the responsibilities of administrative tasks, cleaning, and maintenance should be assigned, or staff should be hired for these functions in supporting the facility.

SAFETY CONSIDERATIONS

There are multiple considerations for safety and layout functionality in facility design. Some include ensuring enough space for individuals to use the facility, proper placement of equipment, and ensuring the facility meets any relevant safety codes and regulations (for example, emergency exits or wheelchair ramps for accessibility). The layout functionality should be well-designed so that traffic can move efficiently with easy access of equipment or workout areas. For example, there should be a minimum of 36 inches for walkway spaces or between squat racks or lifting platforms.

Safety considerations also extend to environmental aspects like proper flooring. For example, some athletic activities require special flooring considerations, such as wooden platforms for weightlifting that have appropriate load-bearing capacity (at least 100 lb/square foot). Adequate lighting and ventilation are additional important safety considerations. For example, light should be bright enough to see clearly without glare (50–100 lumens), and ventilation should be sufficient to keep air circulating and maintained at an optimal temperature range (72–78 °F with humidity no more than 60%).

CONSIDERATIONS FOR MAINTENANCE AND CLEANING

Properly maintaining equipment can reduce long-term costs because the equipment lasts longer without needing to be replaced. Equipment that is durable and easy to repair should be chosen and arranged in a way that allows easy access for maintenance. Regular checks should take place to ensure that equipment is in working order, such as pulleys or cables on weight machines. Many types of equipment require regular cleaning for optimal function (for example, cleaning a treadmill belt or cleaning Olympic-style barbells). It is important to have a master checklist that includes a maintenance and cleaning schedule for each piece of equipment in the facility. In addition, the facility should be designed to make cleaning as efficient as possible. This can include choosing flooring and materials that are easy to clean. For example, carpeted areas are more difficult to keep clean than hard surfaces, so they would not be the flooring of choice in most cases. Particular attention should be paid to regularly cleaning equipment or surfaces that can transfer pathogens through bodily fluids, such as the vinyl pads on weight machines or weight benches.

Considerations for Program and Equipment Needs

Considering program needs requires proactive planning that includes the characteristics of those using the facility. This includes the number of people, training goals, experience, demographics, and scheduling. For example, a facility that plans to have three different collegiate sports teams training each season will need adequate space and scheduling for each team. If there is only one small weight room, it will not be feasible to have all three programs run their training at the same time. As another example, the facility should be able to serve the training goals of the athletes. Sports that need larger amounts of field or court space, such as football, soccer, or basketball, should have practice spaces conveniently located within or beside the facility. Considerations for choosing equipment can include the space available, the budget, the types of workouts or activities in the facility, and the needs and goals of facility users. For example, a facility that is used by collegiate or professional athletes may need more advanced equipment for sports-specific goals (such as Olympic weightlifting bars and plates), whereas a facility for the public might feature more weight machines that require far less technical skill and training to use.

Professional Practice

Scope of Practice

Scope of practice refers to professional qualifications (including legal considerations) that influence the duties and services provided in each role. The NSCA informs this scope of practice by defining the education and certification requirements to be a Certified Strength and Conditioning Specialist (CSCS) and outlining requirements for ethical behavior.

In general, a strength and conditioning professional's scope of practice centers around creating and carrying out safe, effective strength and conditioning programs. This includes understanding and applying physiological principles behind programming, properly conducting and interpreting fitness tests, educating athletes on injury prevention, and providing guidance on aspects like nutrition, recovery, and injury prevention. The scope of practice also includes the ability to individualize programs or exercises to the needs and goals of each athlete.

Activities that fall within the scope of practice may have some general overlap into other allied health domains; however, it is critical to understand how to stay within the scope of practice, both for athlete safety and to avoid legal consequences. For example, it is within the CSCS scope of practice to provide general educational resources like MyPlate to an athlete seeking nutritional guidance but not within the scope of practice to recommend a nutritional supplement.

Codes, Policies, and Procedures Set by the NSCA

Codes, policies, and procedures are used in organizations like the NSCA to fulfill objectives safely and effectively. Main codes set forth by the NSCA include the Professional Code of Ethics, directing how a strength and conditioning professional should conduct themselves to maintain a high standard of practice and avoid legal or disciplinary action. Adhering to ethical guidelines includes maintaining professional conduct with athletes, promoting a safe training environment free of intimidation or mistreatment, and respecting athlete privacy.

As an example of policies and procedures, one of the NSCA's objectives is to use evidence-based information to enhance performance. **Policies** for this include requirements for a passing score on the CSCS certification exam. Ongoing maintenance of continuing education is also required for someone to represent themselves as an NSCA professional. **Procedures** include the methods for administering and scoring the certification exam and how to determine what activities are eligible for continuing education. Individual facilities or programs will have their own policies and procedures, and it is important for the strength and conditioning professional to have awareness and adherence to these as well. Examples could include emergency response policies or procedures for how adolescent athletes should be supervised while training.

Standards and Practices of Relevant Governing Bodies

Strength and conditioning professionals should be aware of all standards and practices of governing bodies that may apply to the athletes they are training. Organizations such as the World Anti-Doping Association (WADA), the U.S. Olympic Committee, and the National Collegiate Athletic Association (NCAA) all have guidelines and regulations that can affect athlete eligibility and participation. For example, each of these organizations has rules on substances that are banned in athletic competitions, and there may be specific guidelines on the nature of medical clearance or eligibility with pre-participation screening. NSCA information highlights the importance of these topics with a general overview, but it is the strength and conditioning professional's responsibility to adhere to all relevant standards and practices for ethical and effective coaching of athletes. This may require seeking out more specific information from relevant organizations, like pursuing continuing education or finding resources to educate athletes on specific regulations.

Recognizing and Responding to Symptoms of Unsafe Training Practices

Some unsafe training practices may be deliberately done by an athlete with the intent of enhancing performance, such as using illegal drugs or performance-enhancing substances or using extreme short-term measures to lose weight. Other unsafe training practices may be ones that an athlete encounters based on their environment or circumstances, such as heat-induced illness or practices with higher potential of overuse injury. Overtraining could be in either category, as an athlete may deliberately do extra training in thinking more is better, or an athlete may experience overtraining from poor programming. It is important for the strength and conditioning professional to proactively educate athletes about the dangers of unsafe training practices.

Regardless of the specific unsafe training practice, responding requires understanding signs and symptoms and monitoring the athlete to determine what action needs to be taken. For example, if an athlete shows signs of heat exhaustion like dizziness and nausea, the athlete should be directed to stop exercising and move to a cooler environment. Medical attention should be the next response if symptoms worsen. Or, if an athlete shows signs of overtraining like fatigue and decreased performance, an appropriate response will include reducing training volume or intensity.

Working with Allied Health Professionals

The main general consideration for utilizing other allied health professionals is in situations that are outside of the strength and conditioning professional's scope of practice. Referring an athlete out or collaborating with other professionals ensures that the athlete will receive appropriate care. For example, if an athlete gets injured during a training session, the strength and conditioning professional would refer the athlete to a physician for diagnosis and treatment. If an athlete discloses signs or symptoms of mental health issues like anxiety or depression, referring them to a psychologist, counselor, or mental health therapist would be necessary. The most effective collaboration with other allied health professionals involves continued monitoring and communication about the athlete's health status while staying within the boundaries of **HIPAA privacy laws**, which prohibit sharing individual medical information without the individual's permission. With the example of an athlete returning from injury and doing rehabilitative exercises, the strength and conditioning professional might have the athlete self-monitor their level of pain and soreness after each training session. This information can then be relayed to the physician to provide further guidelines on progressing the athlete's rehabilitative training plan.

Common Litigation Issues

Informed Consent

Informed consent protects against potential litigation issues by explaining the process, risks, and benefits of an activity to a participant and providing voluntary consent. Often, informed consent is included as part of a form that a participant reads and signs before beginning the chosen activity, ensuring an educated decision about participation. Informed consent typically includes verbiage on **assumption of risk**, which specifically outlines any potential risks associated with the activity. A participant takes on the assumption of risk when they are informed of the risks and voluntarily still chooses to participate.

Using informed consent for every participant shows that reasonable steps were taken to advise participants about the risks and that they had free choice to assent or decline. Let us say a prospective volleyball camp participant reads and signs the informed consent, which explains that training and competing in the sport comes with a risk of injury. If the participant sprains their ankle during training and claims they were not aware of the risks, the informed consent provides legal protection by verifying that the participant had the opportunity to read and understand the risks in their agreement to participate.

Liability Insurance

Liability insurance provides financial protection to professionals against potential lawsuits from injuries or damages that participants may suffer. For example, if a participant gets injured during training and claims the trainer is at fault, liability insurance could cover many of the legal costs if the participant pursues legal action. Depending on the nature and environment of the work, a facility will sometimes provide liability insurance for all staff members. Other times, a strength and conditioning professional will need to purchase their own liability insurance, typically annually or every 2 years.

The **standard of care** is the level and type of care that a competent and skilled professional would provide under similar circumstances. The standard of care depends on the nature of the role, participants, and environment. For example, it is a standard of care for a strength and conditioning professional to account for a participant's current fitness level and medical history in program design. It is also a standard of care to provide clear instruction and supervision during workouts. Lacking adherence to these standards of care increases the risk of participant harm and could lead to litigation issues.

Mitigating the Risk of Litigation Issues

Carefully selecting, maintaining, and accurately using equipment are some key ways to mitigate litigation issues. Equipment should meet industry safety standards, be purchased from reputable retailers, and be appropriate for the users' fitness level and size. Regular inspections should be performed to verify equipment is in good working condition, with any damaged equipment repaired or replaced promptly. The strength and conditioning professional should provide clear instructions and demonstrations on correct equipment use, including proper form and safety precautions. Supervision and safety are other important aspects of equipment use. Supervising participants during the use of equipment allows for any corrections of improper use and quick response to injuries. Equipment should be used and arranged to maximize safety, including not modifying equipment outside of manufacturer instructions and having enough space for use. Not adhering to these could pose legal issues for a strength and conditioning professional. For example, let us say a barbell is labeled by the manufacturer with a maximum weight capacity. If the strength and conditioning professional disregards this information and the excessive load on the barbell injures a participant, this increases the risk of litigation.

NEGLIGENCE

Negligence is a legal concept often used in personal injury lawsuits that describes the failure to act as a reasonably competent and skilled person would act in a given circumstance. There are four elements that constitute a valid negligence claim. **Duty** refers to responsibilities of the role, such as the duty of care to provide a safe training environment. **Breach of duty** occurs when there is a failure to meet the duty of care. For example, failing to instruct a participant on correct equipment use would be a breach of duty. **Proximate cause** involves proving that the breach of duty directly caused the injury. If a participant is injured from incorrect equipment use and it can be proved that they did not receive adequate instruction, this establishes proximate cause. The last element is **damages**, which refers to the harm or injury the participant experiences, which can include not only physical injury but also psychological distress or financial loss. For example, a participant injured due to inadequate equipment use instruction could suffer a bone fracture, which then results in financial loss due to medical expenses and psychological distress from the trauma of the injury.

CSCS Practice Test #1

Want to take this practice test in an online interactive format?
Check out the online resources page, which includes interactive practice questions and much more: **mometrix.com/resources719/cscs-31572**

1. Which of the following athletes is likely to have the highest training volume in their program for resistance training?

a. Marathon runner
b. Bodybuilder
c. Football lineman

2. How can improving flexibility positively impact performance?

a. It speeds up neural transmissions to the brain.
b. It enhances aerobic stamina.
c. It provides the ability to apply force over a greater range of motion.

3. Which of the following is FALSE about fats (lipids)?

a. High levels of high-density lipoproteins (HDL) are associated with increased heart disease risk.
b. The body can store far greater amounts of lipids than carbohydrates.
c. Some amounts of cholesterol are required for bodily functions.

4. The aerobic fitness of two athletes is being compared. If we have a measurement for each of them in mL of O_2 per minute, what needs to be done next to provide an accurate comparison to see who is more aerobically fit?

a. Multiply their scores by the rate pressure product.
b. Add their resting heart rates to each of their scores.
c. Divide their scores by their weights in kilograms.

5. A facility supervisor is deciding where to put a tall cable machine in the layout of their facility. The best place for the machine is:

a. Near an entrance
b. In the middle of the room
c. Along a portion of the wall

6. Which type of injury is significantly more common in female athletes than in male athletes?

a. ACL tear
b. Lumbar vertebrae fracture
c. Lateral ankle sprain

7. What is considered to be one of the reasons caffeine is effective as an ergogenic aid?

a. It enhances the formation of ATP, improving muscular power.
b. It stimulates protein synthesis for greater muscular strength.
c. It increases use of fat as a fuel, sparing glycogen.

8. For optimal safety and function, what should weightlifting platforms be primarily made of?

a. Turf
b. Wood
c. Tile

9. An athlete desires to start using creatine for enhanced performance. What should be considered FIRST before incorporating use of an ergogenic aid?

a. The athlete's method of strength and conditioning and their nutritional habits
b. The athlete's weight for the appropriate creatine dosage
c. The athlete's competition season schedule to structure an appropriate dose and taper of creatine

10. When testing athletes on the 1-RM bench pull, which condition would result in an invalid repetition?

a. The athlete utilizes a pronated grip on the barbell.
b. The athlete's feet are off the ground.
c. The athlete raises the bar 2 inches to the underside of the bench.

11. Teammates are helping each other perform the PNF hamstring stretch. For most effective stretching, what should occur during a passive stretch of the hamstring?

a. Concentrically contracting the quadriceps
b. Isometrically contracting the hamstrings
c. Eccentrically contracting the gastrocnemius

12. A strength and conditioning professional works at a facility that requires injured athletes to have a medical clearance form before returning to training. Such a requirement is an example of:

a. Procedures
b. Policies
c. Standard of care

13. For which type of athlete would complex training be MOST appropriate?

a. Track & field athlete
b. Swimming athlete
c. Skiing athlete

14. Which type of athlete would have the greatest need for considerations of nutrition during their event?

a. A powerlifting athlete
b. A wrestling athlete
c. A long-distance triathlete

15. Which warm-up movements would be MOST appropriate for a plyometric training program?

a. Depth jump and single-leg Romanian deadlift (RDL)
b. A-skip and forward lunges
c. Heel-to-toe walk and static butterfly stretch

16. A strength and conditioning professional wishes to select a dynamic stretch that includes the latissimus dorsi. Which would be the BEST choice?

a. Lunge with overhead side reach
b. Inchworm
c. Straight-leg march

17. Which plyometric drill would be the best for a volleyball player with a training goal to improve their spiking of the ball?

a. 4-hurdle drill
b. Single-leg push-off
c. Backward skip

18. If a training program's goal is to improve force development and force production of the core, which exercise would be the most appropriate?

a. Power clean
b. Curl-ups on an unstable surface, such as a Swiss ball
c. Abdominal crunches using a weight machine

19. The first step in the heart's electrical activity, represented by the P-wave on an ECG, is what?

a. Repolarization of the atria
b. Depolarization of the ventricles
c. Depolarization of the atria

20. Which relaxation technique for improved performance is characterized by an attentional state that focuses on body sensations like warmth or heaviness?

a. Autogenic training
b. Systematic desensitization
c. Attentional control

21. Which of the following would be an example of positive punishment?

a. Having an athlete do five extra minutes of conditioning for being five minutes late to practice
b. Providing a prize for the top-scoring athlete in each season's game
c. Taking away an athlete's team captain status upon observing abusive behavior toward other teammates

22. This athlete is performing a forward step lunge with dumbbells. What correction should be made to the athlete's technique?

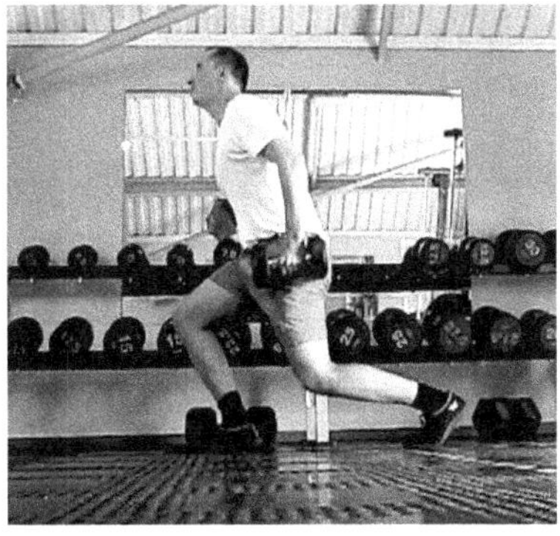

Licensed Under CC BY-SA 4.0 (creativecommons.org/licenses/by-sa/4.0/)
https://commons.wikimedia.org/wiki/File:Jumping_split_squat_with_dumbbells_3.png

a. The lead knee should stay directly over the lead foot.
b. The trailing knee should not be flexed.
c. The torso should be parallel to the floor.

23. The average daily nutrient requirement that is adequate for meeting the nutritional needs of most healthy individuals within a given life cycle is termed the:

a. Recommended Daily Allowance (RDA)
b. Dietary Reference Intake (DRI)
c. Estimated Average Requirement (EAR)

24. For which type of athlete would unilateral training be most suitable?

a. An athlete seeking to develop strength
b. An athlete recovering from injury
c. An athlete whose sport involves movement into the transverse plane

25. Which of the following is the best example of a contraindication?

a. Near-maximal loads are avoided in an athlete's program leading up to the day of competition.
b. Open kinetic chain exercises are avoided for an athlete due to a healing ACL injury.
c. Free weights are avoided for newer athletes, who begin with machines instead.

26. What is the functional component of the neuromuscular system?

a. The motor unit
b. The muscle fiber
c. The myofilament

27. Which sport would be most likely to have a relatively high recruitment of type I fibers and a relatively low recruitment of type II fibers?

a. Marathon running
b. Olympic weightlifting
c. Hockey

28. How does tendon insertion affect force production at a given muscle or muscle group?

a. A tendon insertion closer to the joint center means greater potential force production.
b. Tendon insertion does not have an impact on force production.
c. A tendon insertion further from the joint center means greater potential force production.

29. How high should the box be when performing a barbell step-up?

a. When the foot is on the box, there should be a 90-degree angle at the knee joint.
b. When standing behind the box, the box should come to the midpoint of the athlete's tibia.
c. When standing to the side of the box, it should be level with the top of the athlete's patella.

30. Which of the following would NOT be a positive effect on performance from doing a proper warm-up?

a. Increased core temperature
b. Lowered viscous resistance in muscles
c. Decreased metabolic reactions

31. In an area where physical activity is taking place, relative humidity should not exceed:

a. 60%
b. 50%
c. 70%

32. The picture shown is the ending position for which stability ball exercise?

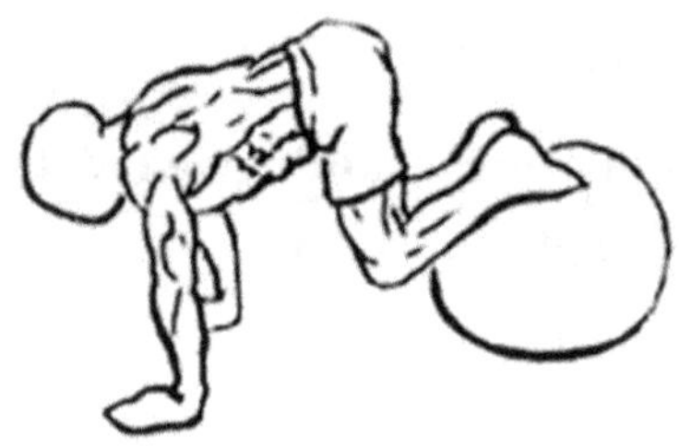

a. Stability ball rollout
b. Stability ball pike
c. Stability ball jackknife

33. Which is an example of an anabolic hormone?

a. Thyroid hormone
b. Insulin-like growth factor (IGF)
c. Cortisol

34. An athlete performs a 1-RM deadlift of 405 lb (184 kg). If this athlete has a strength goal, what is the MOST appropriate load to use for their training program?

a. 315 lb (143 kg)
b. 332 lb (151 kg)
c. 360 lb (163 kg)

35. Which would be most likely to increase the risk of osteoporosis in a female athlete?

a. Presence of the female athlete triad
b. Using multi-joint resistance training exercises
c. Participating in regular resistance training during childhood

36. Assessing the number of foot contacts would be a way to determine the volume of ____ training in order to safely progress over time.

a. agility
b. high-intensity interval (HIIT)
c. plyometric

37. In which technique would observation of vertical displacement be used to ensure an athlete is generating force correctly?

a. Z-drill
b. Y-shaped agility
c. A-skip

38. Of the three types of levers in the body's musculoskeletal system, which one typically has the greatest mechanical advantage?

a. First-class lever
b. Second-class lever
c. Third-class lever

39. Which is NOT part of the five-point body contact position for supine exercises on a bench?

a. Both shoulders are firmly on the bench.
b. Both elbows are firmly on the bench.
c. Buttocks are evenly on the bench.

40. When considering how to build a new facility, what is the minimum recommended amount of space per athlete?

a. 100 square feet
b. 250 square feet
c. 50 square feet

41. Consider the following battery of tests:

Vertical jump
300-yard shuttle
1-RM back squat

For which sport would be these tests be the most appropriate?

a. Wrestling
b. Basketball
c. Rowing

42. A program is being designed for an athlete with strength goals. Which choice of load, reps, volume, and rest periods is best?

a. 67–85% of 1-RM, 1–6 reps, 2–6 sets, and 2–5 minutes of rest in between sets
b. 90–100% of 1-RM, 1–6 reps, 2–3 sets, and 30 seconds of rest or less in between sets
c. 85% or more of 1-RM, 1–6 reps, 2–6 sets, and 2–5 minutes of rest in between sets

43. What are the general recommendations for utilizing carbohydrate loading before an aerobic endurance event?

a. Consume 1.0–1.6 grams of carbohydrates per kilogram of body weight over a 24-hour period before the event.
b. Consume 16 ounces of carbohydrate-containing sports drink in the 2 hours before the event.
c. Consume 8–10 grams of carbohydrates per kilogram of body weight in the three days before the event.

44. Which of the following is NOT a test that measures maximum muscular power?

a. Margaria-Kalamen test
b. Hexagon test
c. 1-RM push jerk

45. Which two minerals warrant particular attention for athletes to ensure they are consuming adequate amounts?

a. Calcium and zinc
b. Magnesium and iron
c. Iron and calcium

46. Where is the barbell's starting position for a hang power clean?

a. On the floor
b. Resting on the anterior deltoids
c. At midthigh or slightly above/below the knees

47. Which structure facilitates activation of the muscle when a change in muscle length is sensed?

a. Golgi tendon organ
b. Muscle spindle
c. Motor units

48. Which best describes the use of progressive-part training in learning the squat clean?

a. Practice multiple variations of the clean in a randomized order, such as the hang power clean and hang squat clean.
b. Practice the squat clean in slow motion with a PVC pipe.
c. Practice power cleans and front squats by themselves, then practice them together as a squat clean.

49. Which is NOT a role of catecholamines?

a. Increasing force production
b. Increasing vasoconstriction
c. Increasing energy availability

50. Which statement about creatine is true?

a. Creatine must be obtained through supplemental forms.
b. Creatine is most effective with a loading dose over a period of days.
c. Creatine tends to promote weight loss due to increasing metabolic rate.

51. An Olympic lifting athlete is consuming a reduced-calorie diet to make their weight class. Which macronutrient will they likely need more of?

a. Carbohydrate
b. Fat
c. Protein

52. Which statement about resistance training programs for youth is true?

a. Youth can expect decreased bone mineral density from training.
b. Youth should not be expected to perform at the same neural skill levels as adults.
c. Youth will improve muscle force production but not muscle mass.

53. An athlete begins to run at a moderate intensity. What will be the primary reason for their increase in ventilation?

a. Increased tidal volume
b. Increased plasma diffusion
c. Increased minute ventilation

54. What would be an example of negligence for a strength and conditioning professional?

a. The strength and conditioning professional forbids an athlete from entering the weightlifting floor due to wearing improper shoes.
b. The strength and conditioning professional allows athletes to bench press unsupervised, and one athlete gets injured.
c. The strength and conditioning professional finds broken equipment, so athletes have to do a circuit for their workout to take turns on the remaining equipment.

55. When would the amortization phase occur in a cycled split squat jump?

a. During the landing in the lunge position
b. During the preparatory countermovement
c. During the explosive phase

56. What type of exercise would be most likely to result in increased mitochondrial density if repeated with training?

a. Cross-country skiing
b. 50 m swim
c. Olympic lifting

57. What is an important consideration in using the 1-RM power clean as a test protocol for athletes?

a. It should not be paired with any other test protocol due to high metabolic demand.
b. It requires a spotter for safety.
c. It is highly technical, so it may not be reliable or valid on an athlete who is inexperienced.

58. Which is NOT a major muscle involved in this movement?

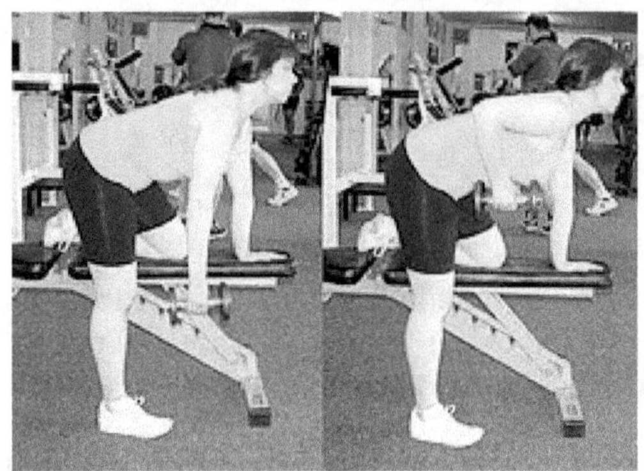

a. Middle trapezius
b. Posterior deltoids
c. Subscapularis

59. A male athlete weighs 63 kilograms and is 1.8 meters tall. In what BMI classification does this athlete fall?

a. Underweight
b. Normal weight
c. Overweight

60. Which of the following is NOT a way to impose the overload principle?

a. Increasing rest periods between sets and exercises
b. Utilizing more complex exercises
c. Adding a second session during one of the week's training days

61. Which of the following is the correct site measurement for obtaining a waist (abdominal) circumference?

a. Three inches below the xiphoid process
b. At the narrowest part of the torso, halfway between the ribcage and the anterior superior iliac crests of the pelvis
c. At the level of the navel

62. A test is performed on an athlete three times within a week, resulting in highly variable scores. This test likely has:

a. Low validity
b. Low reliability
c. Low credibility

63. If two athletes have the same skill level and motivation toward a task, which one will typically be the better performer?

a. The one who has set an outcome goal
b. The one with a desire to avoid failure
c. The one with higher self-efficacy

64. An athlete using a rowing machine first practices the drive of the legs and then practices the pull of the arms. This best describes:

a. Simplification
b. Repetitive-part training
c. Fractionalization

65. Where do most back injuries occur anatomically?

a. Between L4 and L5 or between L5 and S1
b. Between T12 and L1 or between L1 and L2
c. Between T4 and T5 or between C4 and C5

66. A group of male basketball athletes had the following scores for 1-RM testing on the power clean.

Athlete 1: 93 kg (205 lb)
Athlete 2: 98 kg (216 lb)
Athlete 3: 89 kg (196 lb)
Athlete 4: 100 kg (220 lb)

Which statement is INCORRECT?

a. The mean of the scores is 95 kg (209 lb).
b. There is no mode for these scores.
c. The median of the scores is lower than the mean.

67. An athlete is performing a bench press with resistance bands attached at each end of a barbell. Which point in the movement will have the highest resistance load?

a. At the liftoff of the bench press
b. At the lockout of the bench press
c. In the descent phase of the bench press

68. A female volleyball athlete obtains the following scores in testing. What training outcome should be the focus in the athlete's periodized plan going forward?

Pro-agility test: 5.2 seconds
1-RM bench press: 108 lb (49 kg)
Vertical jump: 26 in (66 cm)

a. Improving power
b. Improving strength
c. Improving agility

69. Which modality for older adults would be the most useful for muscular strength and postural stability?

a. Machine-based resistance training
b. Treadmill walking
c. Resistance training with free weights

70. At which phase of movement does the push jerk differ from the push press?

a. In the starting position
b. In the dip of the preparation phase
c. In the catch

71. A coach is targeting the behavior of athletes in cleaning up the weight room after their conditioning sessions through providing praise. This target behavior is termed:

a. Positive reinforcement
b. An operant
c. Enhancing self-efficacy

72. Which substance is released from the sarcoplasmic reticulum to control muscle contraction?

a. Hemoglobin
b. Myosin
c. Calcium

73. Which exercise selection would have the most optimal osteogenic stimuli?

a. Biceps curl and seated chest press
b. Power clean and deadlift
c. Seated calf raise and lying leg curl

74. Which is NOT an effect of resistance training?

a. Increased bone mineral density
b. Increased muscle fiber cross-sectional area
c. Increased blood flow to cartilage

75. An athlete wishes to strengthen their power clean technique. Which exercise would be the best to supplement their training?

a. Romanian deadlift (RDL)
b. Barbell bench press
c. Barbell step-up

76. An athlete in a state championship soccer match has a game in the morning and another game in the late afternoon. Which is the best choice to ensure optimal performance?

a. Consume food or drink that is high in carbohydrates immediately after the first match and at regular intervals throughout the day.
b. Consume approximately 25–50 extra grams of higher-fat foods to preserve lipid stores in the body.
c. Supplement with 2 grams per kilogram body weight of creatine in the 3 days leading up to the soccer matches.

77. Muscles responsible for maintaining posture would have a high composition of which type of muscle fibers?

a. Type I
b. Type IIa
c. Type IIx

78. What type of training program would have the greatest effect on EPOC?

a. High-intensity interval training
b. Aerobic training performed below 50% of VO_2 max
c. Sports-specific dynamic stretching

79. What would be the role of the phosphagen system in a marathon run?

a. It would be less active at the start of the run and then become more active as additional glycogen is needed.
b. It would not be active at all, as a marathon is an aerobic activity.
c. It would be active at the start of the run and then become less active.

80. An obstacle course athlete is training to climb ropes more effectively. Which exercise would be the most appropriate for this goal?

a. Lat pulldown
b. Lateral shoulder raise
c. Flat dumbbell fly

81. An advanced athlete performs a workout with a strength focus on 2 days of the week, a workout with a power focus on 2 days of the week, and a workout with a hypertrophy focus on 1 day of the week. This best describes:

a. Linear periodization
b. Nonlinear periodization
c. Microcycle periodization

82. Which is NOT one of the major muscles utilized in this movement?

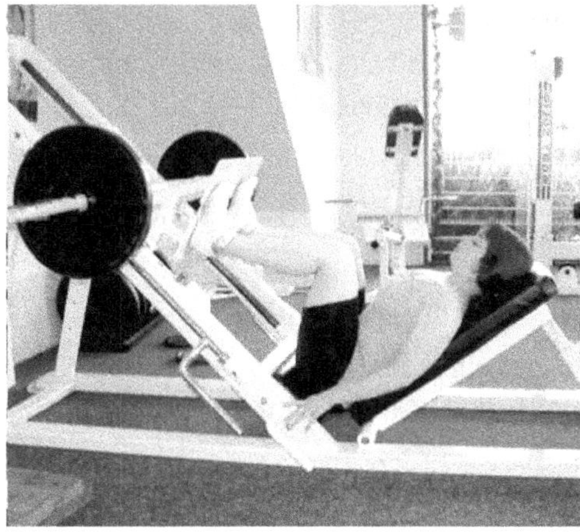

a. Biceps femoris
b. Vastus lateralis
c. Gastrocnemius

83. Which of the following is a closed kinetic chain exercise?

a. Lateral raise
b. Push-up
c. Dumbbell bench press

84. For which type of athlete would it be most suitable to determine the training load using goal repetitions?

a. Distance runner
b. Olympic lifter
c. Professional basketball player

85. Which of the following is INCORRECT in properly spotting an athlete who is performing a barbell bench press?

a. Place the hands in a supinated grip outside the athlete's hands.
b. Keep the hands close to the bar without touching it.
c. Adopt a shoulder-width stance with slight flexion in the knees.

86. Three basic techniques are utilized to flip tires. Which one is pictured?

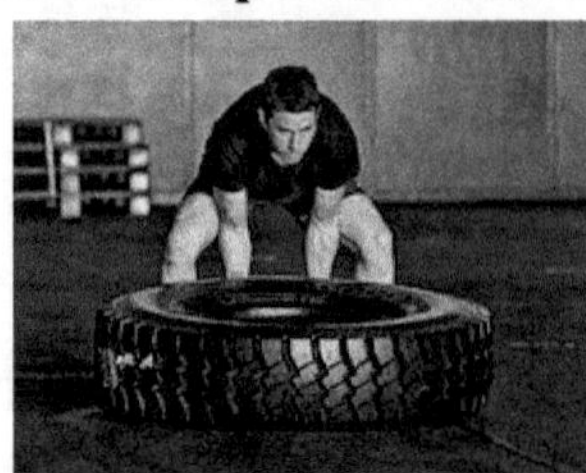

Licensed Under CC BY-SA 3.0 (creativecommons.org/licenses/by-sa/3.0/)
https://commons.wikimedia.org/wiki/File:US_Navy_120206-N-GC412-386_Airman_Mario_Rojas_flips_a_truck_tire_in_the_hangar_bay_while_exercising_aboard_the_Nimitz-class_aircraft_carrier_USS_Jo.jpg

a. Backlift style
b. Sumo
c. Shoulders-against-the-tire

87. A strongman athlete is training with tire flips and log clean-and-press. Which of the following is the MOST appropriate rest period?

a. 1–2 minutes
b. 2–5 minutes
c. 30–90 seconds

88. Which of the following best characterizes bulimia nervosa?

a. Muscle wasting and severe weight loss
b. Recurrent consumption of foods in much smaller amounts than would be customarily consumed
c. Cycles of binging and purging accompanied by feeling a lack of control

89. An athlete is motivated to spend extra time in the weight room because they enjoy the feeling of getting stronger. This best describes:

a. Drive theory
b. Selective attention
c. Intrinsic motivation

90. What is the basis behind using diaphragmatic breathing as a performance-enhancing technique?

a. It allows mental rehearsal of potentially stressful events.
b. It increases parasympathetic activity.
c. It enhances arousal through release of neurotransmitters.

91. Which of the following is an example of a strength and conditioning professional failing to comply with HIPAA guidelines?

a. Providing an athlete with specific supplement recommendations
b. Leaving broken equipment on the fitness floor without an "Out of Order" sign
c. Sharing an athlete's injury report with the rest of the team to provide injury prevention information

92. The head basketball coach at a high school has the junior team watch the varsity team's technique in passing the ball. This is an example of:

a. Observational practice
b. Guided discovery
c. Augmented feedback

93. Which of the following is NOT a sign or symptom of ergogenic aid abuse?

a. Increased sarcopenia
b. Increased liver damage risk
c. Increased blood pressure

94. Which of the following jumps would have the greatest rate of stretch during the eccentric phase?

a. Countermovement jump
b. Approach jump
c. Static squat jump

95. Which of the following plyometric exercises has both a horizontal and a vertical component for the direction of the jump?

a. Depth jump
b. Lateral barrier hop
c. Standing long jump

96. What information must be known about an athlete in order to assign MET values to prescribe exercise intensity?

a. The athlete's maximal oxygen uptake
b. The athlete's resting heart rate
c. The athlete's height and weight

97. Which of the following is an example of a biaxial joint?

a. The elbow
b. The ankle
c. The shoulder

98. An athlete's program is progressing them to utilizing the two-handed kettlebell swing. Which is the best selection of movements that would likely indicate the athlete is ready to progress to the two-handed kettlebell swing if they can perform them correctly?

a. Upright row and push jerk
b. Good morning and bent-over row
c. Hammer curl and abdominal crunch

99. Which is NOT a muscle that is primarily stretched in the spinal twist static stretch?

a. Erector spinae
b. Iliopsoas
c. External oblique

100. An athlete sustained a second-degree lateral ankle sprain five days ago. Which set of movements would be most appropriate to include in their training program?

a. Balance training on wobble board and abdominal crunches
b. Stationary bicycle and single-leg squats
c. Abdominal crunches and stationary bicycle

101. For which type of athlete would eccentric loading in resistance training be most appropriate as a main focus of the training program?

a. Hockey player
b. Rower
c. Long-distance runner

102. Which component is the rate-limiting step in glycolysis?

a. Adenosine monophosphate (AMP)
b. Creatine kinase
c. Phosphofructokinase (PFK)

103. An athlete sustains a partial tear of their anterior cruciate ligament during a soccer match when colliding with the opposing team's goalie. This type of injury is termed a:

a. Sprain
b. Contusion
c. Strain

104. A group of football athletes has finished a periodization cycle for strength and is now entering a periodization cycle for power. How will the assigned volume for the power cycle likely differ from the previous volume for the strength cycle?

a. The volume will be lower.
b. The volume will be dependent on a percent of maximal loads lifted.
c. The volume will be slightly higher.

105. Which of the following is a unilateral movement that would target the rhomboids?

a. One-arm dumbbell bench press
b. Lat pulldown
c. One-arm dumbbell row

106. Cross-country athletes are going through a circuit. The circuit exercises are arranged in the following order. Which choice would be the best fit to go in the blank, based on the existing order?

1. Lunge
2. Vertical chest press
3. Step-up
4. Low-pulley seated row
5. ____________
6. Shoulder press machine

a. Seated leg curl
b. Pec deck
c. Triceps pushdown

107. Which best describes overreaching or functional overreaching (FOR)?

a. Excessive training that results in a long-term decrease in performance
b. Excessive training that results in a short-term decrease in performance
c. Excessive training that results in maintaining performance levels by avoiding high intensities

108. Performing a sit-up requires ____ of the low back in the ___ plane.

a. flexion; transverse
b. extension; sagittal
c. flexion; sagittal

109. What type of carbohydrate molecule is fiber?

a. Monosaccharide
b. Polysaccharide
c. Disaccharide

110. An athlete who participates in intense exercise for hours, such as endurance running or cycling events, and consumes primarily only water is in danger of:

a. Dehydration
b. Iron-deficiency anemia
c. Hyponatremia

111. During a seated leg extension exercise, which muscle is performing a concentric contraction?

a. Semitendinosus
b. Vastus lateralis
c. Biceps femoris

112. The extent of a body's maturation, such as physical growth and development, is called:

a. Chronological age
b. Training age
c. Biological age

113. An athlete is performing a plyometric push-up and has lowered their chest toward the floor as shown. They are now in the position just before explosively pushing off. What would be the name of this phase?

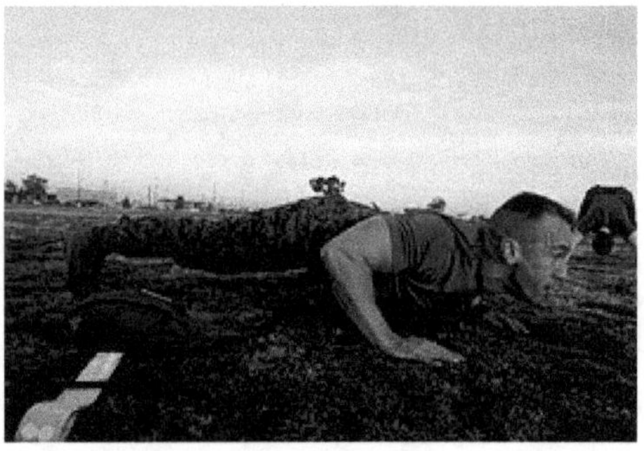

a. Eccentric phase
b. Concentric phase
c. Amortization phase

114. Which statement about reinforcement is true?

a. Only positive reinforcement increases the probability of a given behavior occurring.
b. Use of reinforcement is preferable to punishment.
c. Reinforcement can be used to increase or decrease a given behavior.

115. An athlete performing a power snatch senses that their second pull is not quick enough to get the bar overhead. This is an example of:

a. Augmented feedback
b. Intrinsic feedback
c. Explicit feedback

116. Anabolic steroids are derived from which hormone found naturally in the body?

a. Human growth hormone
b. Epinephrine
c. Testosterone

117. The strength and conditioning specialist for a wrestling team changes up the team's training cycle each month with a new block of exercises. Such a cycle is best described as a:

a. Microcycle
b. Macrocycle
c. Mesocycle

118. Which type of grip is most effective for Olympic lifting movements such as the snatch or clean?

a. False grip
b. Pronated grip
c. Hook grip

119. In the presence of overtraining syndrome (OTS), which of the following would increase?

a. Heart rate
b. Performance
c. Force production

120. The breakdown of carbohydrates (from muscle glycogen or blood glucose) to replenish ATP describes what?

a. Glycolysis
b. Oxidative phosphorylation
c. Gluconeogenesis

121. An athlete reads and signs a form that outlines the nature of participating in fitness testing along with the risks and benefits. This best describes:

a. Informed consent
b. Risk management
c. Waiving liability

122. Which statement about the Valsalva maneuver is FALSE?

a. It can make lifting heavy loads easier.
b. It involves a closed glottis with contracted abdominals and rib cage muscles.
c. It is potentially dangerous due to decreasing blood pressure.

123. An athlete performs a set of pull-ups and then performs a set on the lat pulldown machine. This is an example of:

a. A push-pull exercise order
b. A split routine
c. A compound set

124. Where can a muscle generate the most force, and why?

a. At less than its resting length, because this reduces the joint angle
b. At its resting length, because the maximal number of crossbridge sites are available
c. At more than its resting length, because a longer lever arm means more torque

125. Which of the following situations best describes predictive validity?

a. A coach compares the scores of basketball athletes' anaerobic capacity and agility with the athletes' number of steals and assists per game.
b. A coach administers tests during the midpoint of the baseball season to see if performance has improved from the start of the season.
c. A track coach trains their assistant coaches in a standardized training protocol for all speed assessments.

126. Which macronutrient would be most important during an activity like sprinting?

a. Carbohydrate
b. Protein
c. Fat

127. An athlete who is at beginner-level skill and is asked to perform a complex task will likely have ____ arousal compared to an athlete with greater skill performing the same task.

a. lower
b. higher
c. equal amounts of

128. An athlete is performing a power clean. Where is the best place for the strength and conditioning professional to spot them?

a. The strength and conditioning professional should spot the athlete at the elbows.
b. No spotting is needed.
c. The strength and conditioning professional should spot the athlete at the wrists.

129. What would enhance the reliability of a flexibility assessment for an athlete?

a. Performing a standardized warm-up and standardized stretching before the assessment
b. Performing a set amount of ballistic stretching before the assessment
c. Performing the assessment multiple times throughout the season at varied times of day

130. Which test would be the most appropriate for simulating the needs of the metabolic system in basketball players?

a. 12-minute run
b. 300-yard shuttle
c. Overhead squat

131. Which of the following best describes proper mechanics of the foot strike during high-speed running or sprinting?

a. The midfoot strikes the ground first, and weight is transferred laterally.
b. The heel strikes the ground first, and weight is transferred forward.
c. The ball of the foot strikes the ground first, and weight is transferred forward.

132. Which neurotransmitter is responsible for causing excitation of the sarcolemma and, therefore, muscle contraction?

a. Troponin
b. Action potentials
c. Acetylcholine

133. A strength and conditioning professional is considering using the pro-agility test for assessing a group of hockey athletes. What would be an important consideration for using this test?

a. For the greatest sports-specificity, a test on ice would be preferable.
b. The pro-agility test will not measure change of direction, which is critical for hockey players.
c. The test should be paired with an assessment of maximal strength on the same day for the most valid results.

134. A basketball athlete has mastered the stiff-leg deadlift and the deadlift. Which is the best choice of exercise to progress them to next, based on these movements and the needs of their sport?

a. Hip sled
b. Bent-over row
c. Power clean

135. An athlete sets a goal to perform ten extra minutes of skill work three days a week for the rest of the preseason. This is an example of a:

a. Process goal
b. Psychological goal
c. Outcome goal

136. A sprinter's plan includes high-intensity interval training (HIIT). What intensity will elicit the best training stimulus?

a. 80–85% of VO_2 max
b. 75–80% of VO_2 max
c. 90% or more of VO_2 max

137. Which of the following exercises would NOT be performed inside a typical power rack?

a. Barbell good morning
b. Forward step lunge with barbell
c. Seated barbell shoulder press

138. Which of the following is NOT accurately characterized as a test of local muscular endurance?

a. Maximum distance run in 12 minutes
b. Maximum pull-ups in 1 minute
c. Maximum push-ups to failure

139. A workout is designed for an athlete focused on pushing and pulling movements. Which of the following series of exercises would be the best fit?

a. Bench press, deadlift, calf raise
b. Triceps dip, push-up, lunge
c. Bench press, seated row, pec deck

140. An athlete consuming a meal two hours before a competition should consume approximately __ grams of carbohydrates per kilogram of body weight.

a. 0.5
b. 1
c. 2

141. Which of the following is the correct description of the proper anatomical site to obtain a thigh skinfold?

a. A vertical fold halfway between the hip and knee joints on the anterior portion of the thigh
b. A horizontal fold halfway between the hip and knee joints on the posterior portion of the thigh
c. A diagonal fold halfway between the hip and knee joints on the lateral portion of the thigh

142. Which of the following is NOT part of the axial skeleton?

a. The scapulae
b. The coccyx
c. The sternum

143. Which of the following is the largest contributor to an individual's total energy expenditure?

a. Basal metabolic rate (BMR)
b. Physical activity
c. Thermogenesis

144. Which food would be most suitable for an athlete to consume close to competition time?

a. Mini bagel with fruit
b. Meat and cheese burrito
c. Leafy green and bean salad

145. What would be the most reliable condition for obtaining body mass measurements?

a. In the morning, before intake of food or fluids
b. After a workout
c. At the end of the day, with adequate hydration

146. Which of the following would be the LEAST appropriate training activity for a group of track and field athletes in the preparatory period of periodization?

a. High-repetition resistance training, such as a circuit
b. Sprinting with increased intensity and decreased volume
c. Longer-distance running

147. Which of the following orders of exercises would be the best to maintain good technique and movement quality for an athlete?

a. Bench press, push jerk, lying triceps extension
b. Push jerk, bench press, lying triceps extension
c. Lying triceps extension, bench press, push jerk

148. What is torque as it relates to muscle force?

a. The degree to which a force tends to rotate an object around a specific fulcrum
b. The time rate of doing work
c. The product of muscle force and displacement

149. Which option would be LEAST likely to result in overtraining?

a. Reducing the recovery time during high-intensity interval training
b. Doubling the percent of the training volume
c. Changing the exercise modality from weight machines to free weights

150. Which of the following is a best practice for safety in administering tests?

a. Supervise a cooldown with active recovery after higher-intensity testing.
b. Avoid any practice attempts to reduce fatigue.
c. Perform non-fatiguing tests like body weight or flexibility at the end of the session.

151. An athlete is cleared to return to practice after an ankle sprain. Which of the following tests would be the best choice to assess the stability of each leg?

a. T-test
b. Star excursion balance test
c. Overhead squat

152. In testing maximum muscular strength with a 1-RM, what is the ideal number of attempts after the warm-up?

a. 5–8
b. 1–3
c. 3–5

153. An athlete is performing a log press. What is the most optimal point in the movement for the athlete to exhale?

a. While pressing the log upward
b. Before pressing the log
c. While lowering the log back down to the shoulders

154. In the sliding filament theory, the power stroke of myosin crossbridges comes from the breakdown of what?

a. Calcium
b. ATP
c. Sodium

155. For which training goal would it make the most sense to progress a resistance training program by decreasing the rest period?

a. Strength
b. Power
c. Endurance

156. Athlete A gets excited and pumped up by the cheers of the crowd, while the same cheering makes Athlete B nervous and edgy. The difference here best illustrates which theory?

a. Catastrophe theory
b. Inverted-U theory
c. IZOF theory

157. Movement of the skeletal system is created by which action?

a. Muscles pulling on tendons
b. Tendons pulling on joints
c. Joints pushing on muscles

158. Which of the following is critical for a strength and conditioning professional in order to be a first responder?

a. Having a certification in first aid, CPR, and AED use
b. Having the ability to activate the emergency medical system
c. Having and storing signed waivers for all individuals using the facility

159. Can muscle fiber types change with specific training?

a. No, muscle fiber types are genetically determined.
b. To an extent, some subtypes can change.
c. Yes, any muscle fiber type can change to another type with the right stimulus.

160. Which of the following is NOT a general goal and approach for the fibroblastic repair phase of injury?

a. Prevent excessive muscle atrophy
b. Provide relative rest
c. Provide submaximal exercise

161. Why should mirrors in a facility be placed 20 inches above the floor?

a. To accommodate access for people with disabilities
b. To prevent weights from colliding with the mirror and causing breakage
c. To allow coaches to best see the form of all athletes

162. A training program that does not include adequate rest and variance of training protocol would likely have what main effect on the endocrine system?

a. Increased testosterone production
b. Increased growth hormone production
c. Increased cortisol production

163. The speed of an object plus its direction describes:

a. Acceleration
b. Velocity
c. Power

164. Which of the following would be an example of a superset?

a. Dumbbell bench press and one-arm dumbbell row
b. Deadlift and seated leg curl
c. Back squat and squat box jump

165. Which of the following plyometric exercises does NOT require a countermovement?

a. Jump over barrier
b. Lateral push-off
c. Standing long jump

166. A coach provides their athletes with two choices of skills to work on and whether to do them before or after conditioning drills. This is an example of:

a. Negative reinforcement
b. Extrinsic motivation
c. Self-controlled practice

167. An athlete who consumes a vegan diet asks the strength and conditioning professional about the best way to eat for performance. How can the strength and conditioning professional best help this athlete?

a. Direct the athlete to the MyPlate resource for general guidance.
b. Recommend specific amounts of plant-based foods that are good sources of protein.
c. Encourage the athlete to work with a sports dietitian.

168. The 12-minute run test was used to assess an athlete's strength. This testing situation is best described as:

a. High reliability, high validity
b. High reliability, low validity
c. Low reliability, high validity

169. Which of the following work to rest ratios would be most suitable for a program utilizing interval training?

a. 3:1
b. 1:1
c. 5:1

170. In a periodization program, which of the following would be the best example of supercompensation?

a. An athlete plans to increase their running distance gradually leading up to their next race.
b. An athlete performs successively more difficult plyometric exercises over a period of weeks and improves their sprint speed.
c. An athlete's sleep suffers long-term, and their technique deteriorates as a result.

171. Which of the following is NOT a component of creating a mission statement?

a. The target clientele
b. What makes the service unique
c. The hours and location of the facility

172. An athlete who is new to the back squat is performing it with just a light barbell under the coach's direction. This is an example of:

a. Segmentation
b. Simplification
c. Repetitive-part training

173. Which of the following describes correct posture for the acceleration phase of a sprint?

a. Upright posture with shoulders over hips
b. Slight spinal flexion with neck slightly extended
c. Natural forward trunk lean, head in line with the spine

174. Creating an interval training program to stress the phosphagen system would involve:

a. Long-duration, high-intensity exercise and near-complete recovery between sets
b. Short-duration, lower-intensity exercise and minimal recovery intervals
c. Short-duration, high-intensity exercise and near-complete recovery between sets

175. What happens during the drive phase of utilizing a rowing machine?

a. The hips and knees extend.
b. The torso flexes.
c. The elbows extend.

176. An athlete performs 3 sets of 5 reps of a weightlifting exercise. Based on this, their training goal is most likely for:

a. Endurance
b. Hypertrophy
c. Power

177. An athlete is feeling their heart race and muscles tense in the evening before a championship game. They are likely experiencing:

a. High state anxiety and high arousal
b. Low somatic anxiety and high arousal
c. High trait anxiety and low arousal

178. In which period of the sport season would it be best for a soccer team to develop aerobic endurance?

a. Off-season
b. Preseason
c. In-season

179. A strength and conditioning specialist ensures that the battery of tests for a gymnastics team covers measures of power, strength, and flexibility. This best describes an example of:

a. Test-retest reliability
b. Intra-rater variability
c. Content validity

180. After air enters the trachea during inspiration, where does it pass to next?

a. The bronchi
b. The alveoli
c. The capillaries

181. When considering how to build a new facility, knowing the number of athletes who would use the facility at any given time is critical in order to understand:

a. The scheduling of the staff
b. The choice of equipment selection
c. The traffic flow of the facility

182. Which food is a good source of vitamin C?

a. Fish
b. Oranges
c. Fortified milk

183. A distance running athlete wishes to consume a high GI food before going out for a training run. Which food would be the best choice?

a. White bread
b. Brown rice
c. Milk

184. An athlete on the track team discloses to the strength and conditioning professional that they have been restricting their food and are fearful of gaining weight. How can the strength and conditioning professional best help this athlete?

a. Document the issues and advise the athlete that they may have anorexia.
b. Refer the athlete to a more specifically qualified professional.
c. Provide the athlete with resources on treating and managing disordered eating.

185. Which would NOT be part of a list of job objectives for a strength and conditioning professional?

a. Provide targeted rehabilitation for injured athletes.
b. Develop training programs that take athletes' injury statuses into account.
c. Design strength programs that reduce the likelihood of injuries.

186. What is the role of a synergist in muscular movement?

a. To indirectly assist in movement
b. To act as the prime mover
c. To decelerate the movement

187. Which of the following exercises would benefit most from the use of the Valsalva maneuver?

a. Kettlebell swing
b. Back squat
c. Seated leg curl

188. Which blood pressure response would be most likely during aerobic exercise?

a. Decreased systolic blood pressure, slightly increased diastolic blood pressure
b. Increased systolic blood pressure, slightly decreased or maintained diastolic blood pressure
c. Increased systolic blood pressure, increased diastolic blood pressure

189. Some athletes on the wrestling team have worked to put on sizable muscle mass yet are considering using steroids, as they perceive themselves as looking weak and too small. This situation best describes:

a. Muscle dysmorphia
b. Anorexia nervosa
c. Muscle atrophy

190. Which of the following energy systems is anaerobic?

a. Krebs cycle
b. Glycolysis
c. Electron transport system

191. Muscle hypertrophy occurs due to what biological process?

a. Increased number of myofibrils in the muscle
b. Increased collagen synthesis
c. Increased mitochondrial density

192. What is the proper foot position for the barbell back squat?

a. Heels on floor
b. Wide stance
c. Toes pointed straight forward

193. What are the two arm positions for the front squat?

a. High bar and low bar
b. Parallel-arm and crossed-arm
c. Closed grip and alternate grip

194. In testing a group of athletes, the head coach enforces a standardized rest period between 1-RM attempts, while the assistant coach does not enforce a standardized rest, allowing athletes to perform attempts when they feel ready. This difference describes effects on:

a. Intrasubject variability
b. Inter-rater reliability
c. Discriminant validity

195. In what plane of motion should an athlete be viewed for plyometrics to ensure knees remain midline rather than valgus upon landing?

a. The frontal plane
b. The sagittal plane
c. The transverse plane

196. What would be the best example of using knowledge of performance feedback for an athlete running a 100 m dash?

a. Showing the athlete a video of their running form in slow motion
b. Telling the athlete how quickly they ran the 100 m
c. Having the athlete observe other athletes to compare their form

197. A needs analysis is being conducted for a basketball athlete. Which type of test and corresponding training movements would be most appropriate to the needs of the sport?

a. T-test; hang clean, push press
b. Standing long jump test; stability ball pike, hip sled
c. Star excursion balance test; plyometric chest pass, front and side plank

198. Which of the following correctly lists body composition measurement methods from most valid and reliable to least?

a. Skinfolds; DEXA scan; assessing body weight with a scale
b. Underwater weighing; skinfolds; circumferences
c. Circumferences; skinfolds; DEXA scan

199. An athlete has been tested in a laboratory to assess their specific heart rate and training intensities. What approach would be best for determining the athlete's training intensities?

a. Fick equation
b. Heart-rate reserve
c. Karvonen method

200. What is the primary reason for including an unloading week in a training program?

a. To acclimate to higher training loads during the current training phase
b. To allow the body to recuperate during a week off
c. To prepare the athlete for demands of next training phase

201. What does the Yo-Yo intermittent recovery test assess?

a. Aerobic capacity
b. Maximum muscular power
c. Agility

202. Of the listed choices, which exercise would be most effective for a strength and conditioning professional to use in determining whether a volleyball athlete is ready to begin a plyometric program?

a. Any isometric core variation
b. Any pushing variation
c. Any squatting variation

203. What is combination training?

a. A form of interval training
b. A form of cross-training
c. A form of strength endurance training

204. An athlete has been in a training program for two years and needs to gain significant muscle mass in the upper torso, quadriceps, and hamstrings. What type of training should the strength and conditioning professional use?

a. Upper/lower training split
b. Leg power/upper hypertrophy
c. Total body training

205. A strength and conditioning professional is administering a test battery to a baseball team. What would be the most logical sequence?

a. 1-RM bench press, 505 agility test, skinfolds
b. Skinfolds, 505 agility test, 1-RM bench press
c. 505 agility test, skinfolds, 1-RM bench press

206. Which two variables receive the most attention across the periods of a periodization training plan?

a. Volume and intensity
b. Intensity and exercise selection
c. Frequency and volume

207. In which phase of designing a new facility is a SWOT analysis performed?

a. Design phase
b. Pre-design phase
c. Post-design phase

208. A strength and conditioning specialist is working with a lacrosse team for the first time. After evaluating the needs of the sport, what action is most appropriate to come next?

a. Evaluate the athletes' body compositions and select sports-specific exercises.
b. Evaluate the athletes' training statuses and perform physical testing.
c. Evaluate the athletes' risk for injury by having them perform power exercises.

209. A 43-year-old cycling athlete seeks to train at 65–75% of their target heart rate range. The athlete's resting heart rate is 53. Using the Karvonen method, what is the correct training intensity for this athlete?

a. Approximately 143–165 beats/min
b. Approximately 134–146 beats/min
c. Approximately 115–133 beats/min

210. What sport skill and movement pairing below best exemplifies the specific adaptations to imposed demands (SAID) principle?

a. Free throw shooting; overhead press
b. Freestyle swimming; power clean
c. 100-meter sprinting; barbell row

211. A football team performs the same quick feet lateral agility drill using agility ladders, tires, and then cones. This is an example of:

a. Discovery
b. Segmentation
c. Variable practice

212. A rugby player's 1-RM bench pull from the previous season is 220 lb (100 kg). In retesting their 1-RM, which weight is most appropriate for their first attempt?

a. 132 lb (60 kg)
b. 121 lb (55 kg)
c. 110 lb (50 kg)

213. If an athlete trains aerobically and their body adapts to have a greater stroke volume, what effect will this have on cardiac output?

a. Decreased cardiac output
b. No effect on cardiac output
c. Increased cardiac output

214. The lactate threshold would be ___ in a trained athlete compared to an untrained individual.

a. higher
b. lower
c. the same

215. What is responsible for the bone modeling that increases as a response to resistance training?

a. Hyaline cartilage
b. Osteoblasts
c. Fascia

216. A volleyball player, the team's setter, needs to improve her upper body strength in the off-season training program. What training load and repetition range would a strength and conditioning coach use to bring about the needed improvement in upper body strength?

a. 60–70% load with 4–8 repetitions
b. 70–85% load with 6–10 repetitions
c. 80–90% load with 8–10 repetitions

217. What would be an appropriate primary resistance goal for a lacrosse player in the off-season, which is eight weeks in length?

a. Increasing power clean from 265 lb to 300 lb (120 kg to 136 kg)
b. Increasing bench press from 315 lb to 385 lb (143 kg to 175 kg)
c. Increasing deadlift from 405 lb to 415 lb (184 kg to 188 kg)

218. A distance running athlete is currently running four times per week at an intensity of 65–75% of their target heart rate for 30 minutes each time. Assuming the intensity is kept the same, which is the best choice for the next week's progression?

a. Perform running 3× per week, with each run being 30 minutes.
b. Perform running 5× per week, with each run being 35 minutes.
c. Perform running 4× per week, with 2 runs being 36 minutes and 2 runs being 30 minutes.

219. Using a superset approach in a training program can be most beneficial during what part of the sport season?

a. Postseason
b. Preseason
c. In-season

220. An athlete is performing a training program on the back squat over a period of weeks. If the athlete performs 4 sets of 3 reps, what weight is needed to lift for a volume-load of 2,580 lb (1,170 kg)?

a. 215 lb (97.5 kg)
b. 200 lb (90.7 kg)
c. 195 lb (88.5 kg)

Answer Key and Explanations for Test #1

1. B: Each of the listed athletes has specific needs for their sports or activities that would determine the training goal, whether it is strength, power, hypertrophy, or muscular endurance. An athlete with a hypertrophy goal, such as a bodybuilder, would likely have the highest training volume out of the three, as hypertrophy training usually involves a moderate to high number of reps per set and 3–6 sets per exercise.

2. C: Applying force over a greater range of motion (ROM) increases impulse, meaning the athlete can apply force for longer. Higher flexibility allows athletes to improve their ability to apply force over greater ranges of motion. As an example, if an athlete is sprinting with poor flexibility of the hamstrings, the range of motion over which they can apply force will be smaller than that of a more flexible athlete.

3. A: High-density lipoprotein (HDL) is a protective type of cholesterol that lowers heart disease risk; however, other types of cholesterol—such as low-density lipoproteins (LDL) and triglycerides—are associated with increased heart disease risk when found in high amounts in the body.

4. C: Measuring aerobic fitness is most accurately done through maximal oxygen uptake, which is measured in milliliters of O_2 per kilogram of body weight per minute. Therefore, if our existing measurement is only in mL per minute, the weight of each athlete in kilograms needs to be factored in for a true assessment of each of their aerobic fitness levels.

5. C: Visibility is an important consideration in the layout of a fitness floor and choosing where to put machines. Tall machines are best placed along the walls, like around the perimeter of the space. This leaves the middle of the room more open for coaches or supervisors to see across the space.

6. A: Female athletes are approximately six times more likely to have an ACL tear than male athletes. A well-balanced training program that improves knee strength and control is an important preventative measure.

7. C: Caffeine is thought to improve athletic performance, particularly endurance performance, by increasing fat oxidation through mobilizing free fatty acids. This slows down glycogen depletion, sparing the use of carbohydrates as fuel and thus reducing fatigue.

8. B: Wood platforms are the safest choice for weightlifting movements, as shoes will not slide on them (like they might on tile). It is also important for shoes to not get caught on the platform, which might happen on turf.

9. A: Before utilizing any type of ergogenic aid or sports supplements, an athlete should have an appropriately structured and periodized strength and conditioning program in place and should follow sound nutritional practices. These two aspects are foundational to performance. A supplement will not "solve" things like inconsistent training or inadequate nutrient intake.

10. C: For a valid repetition of the 1-RM bench pull, the athlete must lift the bar high enough to touch the underside of the bench. The other two options describe proper technique for the athlete's setup in this assessment.

11. A: During a passive stretch in PNF stretching, the agonist (the opposite of the muscle being stretched) should concentrically contract to help relax the antagonist (the muscle being stretched, which in this case is the hamstring).

12. B: Policies refer to a facility's rules and regulations, so any type of requirement that a participant or employee must adhere to would be an example of a policy.

13. A: Complex training alternates movements that use the stretch-shortening cycle (like plyometrics) with heavy resistance exercises. This is intended to improve stretch-shortening cycle performance, which is most important in activities that involve rapid changes in velocity like running or jumping.

14. C: Nutrition during an athletic event becomes particularly important when the event is longer than 45 minutes or has multiple events in one day (such as a triathlon). Obtaining adequate nutrients and fluids during the event can ensure the athlete has the best chance of optimal performance. Powerlifting and wrestling are much shorter in duration, so these athletes would not typically need to consume anything during their events.

15. B: Warm-up movements should be at a lower intensity that gradually progresses to mimic the demands of the sport or activity. A-skips and forward lunges fulfill this. The depth jump is itself a challenging plyometric drill and would not be used as part of the warm-up. In addition, static stretches, like the butterfly stretch, are best avoided before activities requiring strength and power.

16. A: The lunge with overhead side reach involves overhead reaching with simultaneous lateral bending, which stretches the latissimus dorsi. The inchworm is a multi-joint exercise that does stretch the latissimus dorsi, but it does not target this muscle as much as the lunge with overhead side reach does. The straight-leg march targets the hamstrings, not the latissimus dorsi.

17. B: The primary jumping needs in volleyball are in a vertical direction. An athlete will have a more powerful and effective volleyball spike if their vertical jump to meet the ball is also effective. The single-leg push-off is the only listed choice that involves vertical jumping and thus is most directly applicable to volleyball.

18. A: Using an unstable surface can reduce the rate of force development required during the exercise, so choice B would not be most suitable for this goal. While choice C would isolate the core, there is no evidence that isolating it would improve performance; however, as a power clean is a free weight activity that requires rapid force generation, it would be most effective for the program's goal in activating core musculature in this manner.

19. C: The P-wave occurs when cardiac muscle cells change electric potential, causing depolarization of the atria, which is the first step in the heart's electrical activity. Depolarization of the ventricles occurs in the second step, represented by the QRS complex on an ECG. Repolarization of the atria also occurs during this second step, but its waveform is not typically apparent on an ECG due to being hidden by the QRS complex.

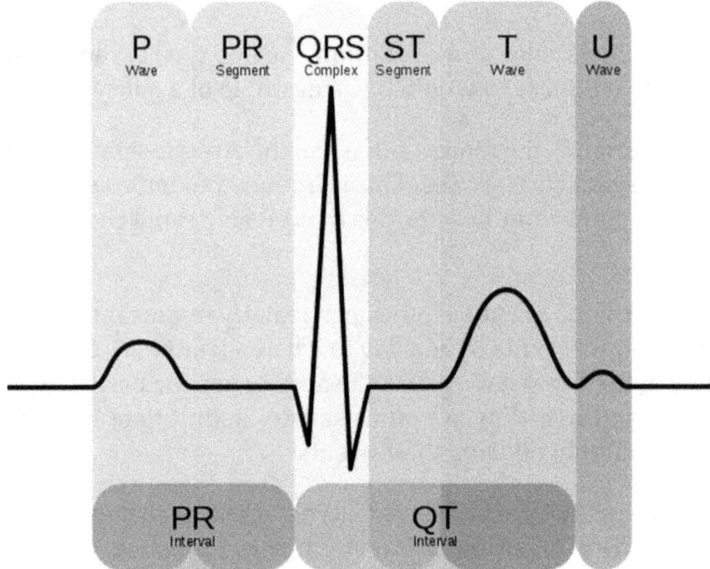

20. A: The relaxation technique of autogenic training has similarities to progressive muscular relaxation, but rather than going through cycles of tensing and relaxing, autogenic training places the attentional focus solely on body sensations, such as sensing heaviness, without using tension.

21. A: In positive punishment, something is presented that is intended to decrease the occurrence of a given behavior, or operant. The coach is presenting the athlete with the penalty of requiring extra conditioning, which is intended to decrease the likelihood that the athlete will be late again in the future.

22. A: In this image, the athlete's lead knee is significantly over the lead foot. This shifts the weight to being too far forward over the knee, rather than evenly balanced between the lead foot and the trailing foot.

23. A: DRIs are overarching sets of nutrient intakes, while the RDA is a *type* of DRI. The EAR describes the average daily nutrient intake that is considered sufficient to meet half of a given healthy population's needs.

24. B: Unilateral training works one side of the body at a time. It is best utilized for helping to reduce bilateral asymmetries or rehabilitating an injured athlete to ultimately promote more balanced, bilateral movement.

25. B: A contraindication is an injury or condition that makes a given movement or practice inadvisable, with the assumption that such an action would make the injury or condition worse. Simply avoiding an exercise or movement is not a contraindication, as there may be other logical reasons for doing so, like in options A and C.

26. A: The motor unit activates muscle fibers, using signals from the alpha motor neuron to dictate firing rate or frequency. Myofilaments, like actin and myosin, are components in a muscle fiber that interact for muscle contraction.

27. A: Type I fibers are termed *slow-twitch fibers*, as they have a high aerobic capacity and are more resistant to fatigue. High relative involvement of type I fibers is found in longer-duration, lower-intensity activities, like marathon running. Olympic weightlifting and hockey are sports that require rapid force development and high power output, so they would have relatively high involvement of type II fibers instead.

28. C: When a tendon is inserted further from the joint center, this creates a longer moment arm for muscle force to act. For example, the presence of a patella allows the quadriceps tendon to be further from the knee joint, improving its mechanical advantage.

29. A: Having a 90-degree angle at the knee joint when stepping on the box ensures that it will be high enough to activate the major muscles of the lower body but not so high that the athlete will have difficulty stepping on it.

30. C: A proper warm-up has many physical effects on the body, and the effect on metabolism is to increase metabolic reactions. One way to think of this is that warming up allows us to use energy more efficiently, boosting metabolism.

31. A: Relative humidity should not exceed 60%, as anything higher than that can encourage growth of bacteria, leading to potential spread of infections among participants.

32. C: The stability ball jackknife begins in a quadruped position with feet on the ball and hands placed on the floor. Unlike the pike, which keeps the legs straight to pull the ball in, the jackknife is performed by flexing the hips and knees to bring the ball closer to the chest, then returning to the start position.

33. B: The role of anabolic hormones is to promote tissue building, of which IGF is one example, along with others like testosterone. Thyroid hormone is a permissive hormone, letting other hormones' actions happen, and cortisol is a catabolic hormone involved in the breakdown of proteins.

34. C: Load can be expressed as a percent of 1-RM, where the percent range is based on the training goal. For a training goal of strength, a load of 85% or greater of 1-RM is recommended. Multiplying the athlete's 1-RM of 405 by 0.85 yields a number of 344 lb (156 kg). The athlete would need to use a load that is at least this heavy. The other two choices are under the 85%.

35. A: The female athlete triad is characterized by long periods of training during which caloric intake is insufficient and menstrual function ceases. Lack of adequate energy intake and hormonal effects can make osteoporosis more likely due to decreased bone mineral density.

36. C: Plyometric training's volume is assessed through the number of foot contacts (or catches/throws if upper body movements are performed). Keeping these volumes to the general guidelines for beginner, intermediate, or advanced athletes ensures a proper training load.

37. C: In the A-skip, the objective is to actively drive the swing leg down to the ground while the opposing leg then pops up. This force generation results in vertical displacement. The other two techniques involve change of direction and rapid acceleration and deceleration rather than horizontal movement.

38. B: A second-class lever typically has the greatest mechanical advantage because the presence of a long moment arm means that the muscle force can overcome the resistive force. First-class and third-class levers typically have a mechanical disadvantage because the resistive force is greater than the muscle force.

39. B: The five-point body position allows stability and support for supine exercises like the bench press; however, the elbows do not need to be firmly on the bench, as they should be free to move during such an exercise.

40. A: One hundred square feet per athlete is the recommended amount of space for optimal safety and function within the facility.

41. B: This array of tests is most specific to basketball, as vertical jumping is required, anaerobic capacity is needed, and muscular strength from the legs is also important. While a case could potentially be made for one or two of these tests being applied to the other choices, neither wrestling nor rowing typically involves jumping, ruling each of them out.

42. C: The goals of strength, hypertrophy, and endurance are all distinctive. A strength goal requires the longest rest but the heaviest load as a percent of 1-RM. Choice A has the correct reps, sets, and rest for a strength goal, but the load is incorrect because 67–85% of 1-RM is suited for muscular hypertrophy. Choice B's main issue is the rest period—30 seconds or less would be unrealistic for safely working toward a strength-based goal at high levels of 1-RM.

43. C: Carbohydrate loading through consuming 8–10 grams of carbohydrates per kilogram of body weight in the three days before an aerobic endurance event can maximize glycogen stores, reducing fatigue from glycogen depletion.

44. B: The hexagon test measures agility, not maximum muscular power. Any 1-RM explosive movement, of which the push jerk is one example, will measure muscular power, and the Margaria-Kalamen test is designed specifically to measure muscular power.

45. C: Failure to consume enough calcium and/or iron can have implications for impaired performance. As iron is needed for oxygen transport, an iron deficiency can lower performance. As calcium is needed for bone density and bone mass, not consuming enough can compromise structural integrity of the bones and increase bone fracture risk.

46. C: In the hang power clean, the bar begins at midthigh or slightly above or below the knees. After the bar is initially lifted from the floor for this variation on the power clean, it does not touch the floor again until the repetitions are complete.

47. B: Both the muscle spindle and the Golgi tendon organ are types of proprioceptors, which can sense tension in the muscle length; however, only the muscle spindle functions to activate the muscle when a change in length is sensed. The Golgi tendon organ has the opposite function, inhibiting muscle activation when a change in length is sensed.

48. C: Progressive-part training is useful when a skill is complex or has multiple parts. A squat clean involves both a clean and a squat, and these can be separated into two clear parts. Progressive-part training can be used to practice each part in isolation before putting them together.

49. B: Catecholamines, like epinephrine, stimulate a fight-or-flight response. Levels of catecholamines increase in the body in response to stress, including the physical stress of exercise. Catecholamines are important for acute strength and power, so increased vasodilation to get more blood flow to the working muscles is one of their roles, not vasoconstriction.

50. B: Because creatine's method of effectiveness as an ergogenic aid relies on energy metabolism and increasing stored creatine in the muscles, it is best taken over a period of days, such as five days of a loading dose. The other choices are false, as creatine occurs naturally in meat and fish, and creatine tends to promote weight gain due to increased total body water.

51. C: Consuming higher amounts of protein relative to caloric intake can help to preserve lean muscle if someone is choosing to eat less for a weight loss goal.

52. B: In youth, the nervous system may still be undergoing development, meaning that movements may lack speed or skill. Therefore, youth should not be treated as "small adults" and should have individualized training programs that meet their needs.

53. A: Tidal volume is the amount of air inhaled and exhaled with each breath and is the primary cause for ventilation increase during low- to moderate-intensity exercise. Minute ventilation, or the volume of air breathed per minute, does play a role, but it does not start to rapidly increase until higher intensities of exercise.

54. B: Negligence is the failure to act as a reasonable and prudent person would act under similar circumstances. In this case, a strength and conditioning professional's responsibility is to adequately supervise athletes, so failure to uphold this responsibility is acting in a negligent manner.

55. A: As the amortization phase occurs between the eccentric and concentric phases, in the cycled split squat jump, it would occur as the athlete lands in the lunge position and movement briefly stops. Proper technique to maximize plyometric effects would require that the athlete keep the length of time in this landing position as minimal as possible.

56. A: Mitochondria increase in density as an adaptation to aerobic training, which allows the working muscles to uptake and utilize more oxygen. Cross-country skiing is primarily an aerobic activity of longer duration and lower intensity, while the other two choices are high-intensity, short-duration and primarily anaerobic in nature.

57. C: Athletes who are novices or inexperienced in a given movement or test protocol are not typically good candidates for a valid or reliable assessment. For example, an athlete who does not know how to perform the power clean accurately may obtain a score indicating low strength, while this result is more from poor technique versus a true lack of strength.

58. C: The one-arm dumbbell row does not target the subscapularis, which is part of the rotator cuff muscles and is most active during movements that involve some type of rotation (such as internal or external) at the shoulder joint.

59. B: Body mass index, or BMI, is calculated as weight in kilograms divided by height in meters squared.

$$\frac{63\text{ kg}}{(1.8\text{ m})^2} = 19.4$$

In BMI classifications, this number falls within the normal range, which is 18.5–24.9.

60. A: The overload principle involves imposing a more intense stimulus to stress the body at higher levels than it's used to. Increasing the rest is the only choice that would make a given workout or training program less intense.

61. C: The navel, also known as the umbilicus or belly button, provides an anatomical landmark for an individual's waist circumference. It allows reliable measurements because it is visible and consistent for a given individual.

62. B: A test that is reliable has a high degree of consistency or repeatability. Testing an athlete and getting highly variable scores suggests low reliability and could indicate that this test's results are not very meaningful to actually analyze performance improvements.

63. C: High self-efficacy for a given situation means that someone perceives that they have the abilities to perform. Self-efficacy can set one athlete above another, as skill and motivation are not enough to promote self-belief.

64. C: Fractionalization as a practice technique is characterized by breaking a task into components that normally would occur simultaneously. In this case, a rowing machine uses both the legs and arms at the same time, but this practice technique has the athlete performing each of them independently.

65. A: Most back injuries occur between the lowest two lumbar vertebrae (L4 and L5) or between the lowest lumbar vertebra and sacral vertebra (L5 and S1). The discs associated with these vertebrae have very high compressive forces and high levels of torque during loading.

66. C: The calculated mean is accurate, and each score appears only once, making a mode nonexistent; however, the calculated median of the scores (the average of the two middle-most scores) is 95.5 kg or 210 lb, which is slightly higher than the mean.

67. B: Using bands as external resistance to a weighted exercise, such as the bench press, will mean that the maximal amount of resistance is wherever the topmost position of the barbell occurs in the movement, typically the lockout. At the lockout of the bench press, the bands will be stretched to their greatest extent, thus providing the greatest stretch resistance.

68. C: This athlete has obtained scores near the top of the percentiles for the bench press and vertical jump; however, her score for the pro-agility test is low (between the 20th and 30th percentile). Therefore, improving her agility would be the priority out of the three options.

69. C: Free weights provide the most direct training stimulus for muscular strength and postural stability. While machines can be used, they will not provide the same level of adaptations. Treadmill walking is a useful form of exercise for the cardiovascular system but would not be the most useful choice for developing strength.

70. C: The push press and push jerk have the same starting position and dip; however, the push press catch position is with the body fully extended, and the push jerk catch position is with the hips and knees in a dipped (slightly flexed) position.

71. B: A target behavior, or operant, is one that is manipulated to increase the probability of a desirable outcome or decrease the probability of an undesirable outcome. In this case, the coach is praising the athletes for cleaning up the weight room, making the cleaning behavior (the operant) more likely to happen in the future.

72. C: Hemoglobin's primary role is to transport oxygen in the blood, not to directly contribute to muscle contraction. Myosin is a type of myofilament that pairs with actin to form crossbridges during muscle contraction, so it plays an important role in muscle contraction but is not a stored substance that gets released. The release of calcium from the sarcoplasmic reticulum is the first step in the sliding filament theory of muscle contraction.

73. B: Exercises that promote osteogenic stimuli stimulate formation of new bone by overloading the bone with appropriate stress. The best choices for this training adaptation are movements that are multi-joint and direct forces through the structure of the skeleton. The other two choices are single-joint and/or machine-based and would be less effective at forming new bone growth.

74. C: Resistance training can boost movement of nutrients to cartilage and prevent it from undergoing atrophy, but as cartilage does not have a blood supply, resistance training would have no effect on blood flow specifically to cartilage.

75. A: The Romanian deadlift (RDL) closely mimics the transition phase of the power clean as the bar rises just above the knees. Utilizing the RDL would best build strength and proper technique as the athlete goes into the second pull. While the other choices would build strength, they do not have similar movements to the power clean.

76. A: The primary nutritional goal of this athlete based on their sport and needs is to have adequate recovery between the soccer games. The demands of playing one game and needing to play a second game within the same day are likely to deplete muscle glycogen. Consuming foods or drinks high in carbohydrates after the first game and at regular intervals will increase muscle glycogen stores and reduce fatigue for the second game.

77. A: Muscles responsible for maintaining posture would be more fatigue-resistant and need to contract at low intensities over long periods of time. This description characterizes type I slow-twitch fibers.

78. A: EPOC, or excess postexercise oxygen consumption, occurs after exercise as the body continues to use oxygen to restore itself back to resting values. Exercise intensity plays the largest role in EPOC. Higher intensities will elicit greater EPOC values. As the other two choices are not high in intensity, they are unlikely to elicit a significant amount of EPOC.

79. C: The phosphagen system's primary role is to fuel high-intensity, short-duration exercise. It derives its fuel from creatine phosphate and ATP hydrolysis, not glycogen breakdown; however, all energy systems are active at any given time, though their involvement depends on the nature of the exercise's intensity and duration. Regardless of the activity, the body's oxygen deficit means that energy is first supplied anaerobically, as the aerobic system responds more slowly.

80. A: In analyzing the needs of the rope climb movement, it is primarily a pulling movement that requires strength from the muscles of the upper and middle back. Therefore, a lat pulldown would be most effective, as it works those muscles.

81. B: Nonlinear periodization, also termed daily undulating periodization, involves large daily variance in the load and volume of exercises performed.

82. C: The hip sled exercise works the major muscles of the quadriceps group, the hamstring group, and the gluteus maximus; however, it does not primarily work the gastrocnemius, the major calf muscle in the lower leg.

83. B: In a closed kinetic chain exercise, the distal segment(s) are stationary. A push-up is an example of an upper body closed kinetic chain exercise, as the hands are affixed to the floor to perform the exercise.

84. A: Using goal repetitions for training load means that the athlete does not need to perform a 1-RM. Maximal strength is not warranted for the needs of a distance runner. Therefore, a method like finding a 12-RM or a 15-RM and having the athlete train to reach that amount of repetitions would be more useful for this athlete.

85. A: Proper spotting of a movement such as the barbell bench press should have the hand placement in an alternated grip with hands inside the athlete's hands.

86. B: In the sumo technique, the athlete adopts a wide stance where the feet are significantly wider than hip-width and the arms are inside of the stance with a narrower grip.

87. B: The nature of this athlete's activities means that the training goal is strength/power. This means the athlete is lifting heavy loads and needs more rest for safe and successful completion of the movements. Having rest that is too short may compromise form and technique.

88. C: Bulimia nervosa is characterized by recurrent consumption of foods in significantly greater amounts than would normally be consumed (the opposite of option B), also known as binging or binge eating; however, bulimia is distinct from binge eating disorder because individuals then feel compelled to purge food in some way, such as vomiting. These cycles of binge eating and purging provoke feelings of being out of control. Choice A describes anorexia. Individuals with bulimia are typically normal weight, not underweight.

89. C: An individual with high intrinsic motivation for a given activity is motivated from within—that is, they find the activity inherently rewarding and enjoyable.

90. B: Diaphragmatic breathing is used to promote a relaxation response. The deep and rhythmic breathing decreases the fight-or-flight response of the sympathetic nervous system, conversely increasing the activity of the parasympathetic system.

91. C: HIPAA, or the Health Insurance Portability and Accountability Act, is a federal regulatory law that covers the protection and privacy of individual participants' health care information. The details in an injury report are confidential information that should not be shared without written authorization. The strength and conditioning professional could instead share basic injury prevention guidelines without providing any identifying information that links back to the affected athlete.

92. A: Observational practice involves watching the skill or task, whether through other persons, videos, etc. The intent is that watching skills being performed helps improve one's own motor skills.

93. A: Ergogenic aids, such as anabolic steroids, are associated with a variety of side effects. Some ergogenic aids can result in mood swings, increased aggression and arousal, liver damage, and hypertension. Sarcopenia is a loss of muscle mass and strength, often associated with the aging process, while ergogenic aids are typically used to increase muscle mass or strength.

94. B: The approach jump has the greatest rate of stretch during the eccentric phase and thus results in the highest jump height. This jump uses the quickest and most forceful eccentric phase out of the answer choices, meaning the most power can be generated.

95. B: The depth jump has only a vertical component, and the standing long jump has only a horizontal component; however, the lateral barrier jump involves not only jumping high enough to clear the barrier vertically but jumping to the side enough (horizontally) to land on the other side of the barrier.

96. A: An MET, or metabolic equivalent, is equal to 3.5 mL per kg of oxygen consumption, the amount of oxygen the body requires at rest. Thus, in order to use METs for intensity, the maximal oxygen uptake must be known so that there is an upper range based on the individual's abilities.

97. B: Biaxial means that the joint has movement around two perpendicular axes. This rules out the elbow, as it is a hinge joint with one axis. It also rules out the shoulder, which can move freely around multiple axes because it is a ball-and-socket joint. The ankle is the only choice that allows movement around only two axes.

98. B: Proper form for the two-handed kettlebell swing includes flexing at the hips while keeping the spine in a neutral position. The good morning and the bent-over row would both mimic a portion of the kettlebell swing's movement, so an athlete performing these correctly would be a good indication that they may be ready for the kettlebell swing.

99. B: The spinal twist involves a seated lateral rotation with one leg crossed over the other. As the iliopsoas works primarily to flex the spine and the hip, it would be stretched with some type of hip extension or spinal extension movement instead.

100. C: This athlete's injury is relatively recent, so they are in the inflammatory response phase, when resting the affected area is needed to minimize further inflammation. While the athlete is not yet ready to load the healing tissue with a movement like a single-leg squat or wobble board balance training, the athlete can maintain their fitness in other ways that utilize other muscle groups or do not directly load the injured area.

101. A: Eccentric strength is particularly important for activities that require agility—rapid change of direction. Such training allows the neuromuscular system to adapt to decelerating the body appropriately. The other sports listed besides hockey do not involve rapid changes of direction.

102. C: PFK is one of three important glycolytic enzymes that control the process of glycolysis. The reaction that it controls allows cells to metabolize glucose over storing it as glycogen. AMP is a byproduct of ATP hydrolysis, and creatine kinase is a catalyst that synthesizes ATP.

103. A: The term *sprain* describes trauma to a ligament of the body, and it has three degrees depending on severity. The other terms describe types of trauma to a muscle.

104. A: Training for power typically involves complex movements that require technical skills, such as the snatch or the clean and jerk. To emphasize the quality of power movements, the volume is typically lower than the volume in training for strength due to lighter loads and fewer repetitions.

105. C: Unilateral movements work only one side of the body at a time, ruling out the lat pulldown. The rhomboids are targeted in rowing or pulling movements. The bench press does not primarily target them, as it is a pushing movement.

106. A: The existing order of the circuit alternates lower body exercises with upper body exercises. Therefore, the most logical choice for the blank is to select a lower body exercise, since an upper body exercise is before and after it.

107. B: Overreaching, or functional overreaching (FOR), is a temporary, short-term response to training overload. While too much overreaching can lead to overtraining, it can be a valid part of training programs to overload the body as long as it is well managed.

108. C: Flexion of the spine is done during movements that involve bending forward, ruling out extension. The transverse plane slices the body into upper and lower sections. Movements occurring in this plane involve rotation. As a sit-up is not a rotational movement, this rules out the transverse plane.

109. B: Polysaccharides are complex carbohydrates, such as fiber, glycogen, and starch, built from several molecules of sugar. Monosaccharides are single-sugar molecules, like fructose. Disaccharides are two-sugar molecules, like sucrose.

110. C: Hyponatremia is a dangerous condition resulting from dilution of blood sodium levels. This may occur when an athlete is losing large amounts of sodium in sweat but is not adequately replenishing the sodium. In this situation, drinking only water is likely not enough to replace the sodium lost in sweat, and the athlete should consume sodium-containing foods or beverages, such as a sports drink.

111. B: A seated leg extension exercise involves a concentric contraction of the quadriceps, since straightening the legs against resistance shortens this muscle group. The vastus lateralis is the only listed choice that is one of the quadriceps muscles. The semitendinosus and biceps femoris are part of the hamstrings.

112. C: Of the incorrect choices, chronological age is simply one's numerical age in months or years. Training age is the amount of time that a formal, supervised training program has been followed.

113. C: The amortization phase in plyometric movements is the time between the eccentric and concentric phases. Here, the athlete has completed the eccentric lowering and is just about to enact a concentric, explosive action for the plyometric portion of the push-up. The amortization phase must be kept short to best maximize activity of the stretch reflex.

114. B: While both reinforcement and punishment can be used by a strength and conditioning professional or coach, reinforcement is preferable because it focuses on what should be done or is being done well. Reinforcement can be positive or negative, and both are used to increase the frequency of a desired behavior, ruling out option A and option C. Punishment can also be positive or negative, but it is used to decrease the frequency of a desired behavior.

115. B: Intrinsic feedback comes from within, generated by an athlete's own senses—as opposed to other types of feedback, like augmented feedback, that come from an external source, like a coach or a video.

116. C: Anabolic steroids are a synthetic version of testosterone. Testosterone by itself is not an effective ergogenic aid due to rapid degradation, so using it as an ergogenic aid requires that it be modified into human-made versions, which provide testosterone in levels exceeding what the body would make naturally.

117. C: A periodization cycle lasting 2–6 weeks is called a mesocycle. A macrocycle is longer, lasting months to a year, and a microcycle is smaller, lasting a few days to two weeks.

118. C: In the hook grip, the thumb is underneath the index and middle finger, which is the main differentiator from the pronated grip. This hand position allows a strong position for movements requiring high levels of power, like Olympic lifts.

119. A: OTS is a long-term performance decrease that can result in many body system disturbances, causing undesirable effects like decreased force production. An increased heart rate at rest can indicate that the body is overtraining and not recovering adequately.

120. A: Glycolysis allows stored glycogen or glucose to be used as fuel through breaking it down. Oxidative phosphorylation describes resynthesizing ATP as part of the electron transport chain. Gluconeogenesis is when glucose is formed from noncarbohydrate sources.

121. A: When a participant is fully informed (whether verbally or through reading a form) about the risks and benefits of an activity and is permitted to choose whether to participate or not, this describes informed consent.

122. C: The Valsalva maneuver does have potential danger associated with blood pressure, such as the risk of blacking out, but this is due to the muscle contraction and closed glottis increasing blood pressure, not decreasing it.

123. C: Both pull-ups and lat pulldowns target the same general muscle group: the latissimus dorsi and the rhomboids. When an individual performs two sequential exercises for the same muscle group, this is called a compound set.

124. B: A muscle at resting length has the actin and myosin filaments—important components of muscle contraction—next to each other, forming the greatest number of crossbridge sites. A contracted (shortened) muscle or a lengthened (stretched) muscle means there is less overlap between these sites, meaning less potential force production.

125. A: Predictive validity describes the extent to which a test score aligns with (or predicts) future performance. In the situation presented in answer A, the coach is assessing if the test scores are transferring into real-life performance in game play.

126. A: Sprinting would be an anaerobic activity because it requires a high power output and rapid muscle contraction speed. Carbohydrate is the only listed choice that can be metabolized without oxygen, making it most critical during an anaerobic activity.

127. B: Arousal is influenced by many factors, but skill level and task complexity are two important ones. A more skilled athlete typically can perform the same task with lower arousal compared to a less skilled athlete.

128. B: Power exercises, such as a snatch or clean, should not be spotted. The explosive nature of these movements can result in injury to the spotter and/or the athlete. When an athlete fails one of these lifts, they should allow the weight to fall to the platform and move out of the way.

129. A: As reliability is the measure of consistency of a test, the more standardized the pre-testing procedure is, the more it will contribute to consistent assessment. Ballistic stretching should not be permitted during flexibility testing, as it has a higher risk of injury over benefits.

130. B: The 300-yard shuttle test is the most appropriate because it measures anaerobic capacity. In basketball, the needs of the metabolic system are primarily for 30–90 second, start-and-stop bursts of speed.

131. C: During high-speed running or sprinting, athletes contact the ground on the forefoot (ball of the foot) with the foot landing under or near the body's center of mass to reduce braking forces and allow rapid force production.

132. C: While all of these play a role in muscle contraction, acetylcholine is the only listed choice that is a neurotransmitter. Troponin is a protein that binds with calcium in its role in muscle contraction, and action potentials are electrical impulses that release calcium to enable muscle contraction.

133. A: While agility is an important skill for hockey players and the pro-agility test does measure change of direction, performing a test that involves sprinting on land will be less sports-specific to emulating the needs of hockey.

134. C: The power clean would be the most logical continuation in progressing to a more complex movement, as the deadlift closely resembles the transition phase needed in the power clean, and power is a primary need in basketball. While the other two choices could be viable for building strength, they are a less logical progression from the movements the athlete has already mastered.

135. A: Process goals are focused on action and effort. In this case, the athlete can measure success by the frequency with which they adhere to this regular behavior.

136. C: HIIT training requires intensities at 90% or more of VO_2 max to properly challenge the anaerobic glycolysis system. HIIT may use durations of 45 seconds up to 4 minutes to elicit such stimuli.

137. B: The forward step lunge with barbell cannot be performed inside of a typical power rack, as the nature of the lunge movement means that the athlete's barbell would collide with the rack structure; however, a rack with supports on the outside could be utilized.

138. A: Tests of local muscular endurance require certain muscle groups to perform repeated contractions against submaximal resistance. The 12-minute run is more accurately characterized as a test of aerobic capacity because it is full-body and includes the cardiovascular system, not just localized to specific muscle groups.

139. C: The other two choices have at least one movement that is not a push/pull movement, such as lunges or calf raises. Only choice C solely comprises pushing/pulling movements.

140. B: This amount is likely to provide enough carbohydrates to maximize blood glucose and glycogen while not requiring the athlete to consume overly large amounts of food a few hours before competing.

141. A: It is important to understand both the anatomical landmarks and the direction for each skinfold, such as the description for the thigh skinfold, as performing a skinfold improperly would compromise the validity of a body composition measurement.

142. A: The axial skeleton comprises the skull, all vertebrae from the cervical vertebrae down to the coccyx, the sternum, and the ribs. All other bones, including the scapulae, are part of the appendicular skeleton.

143. A: Basal metabolic rate contributes about 65–70% of an individual's total energy expenditure. Out of an individual's total calorie needs per day, the majority of these calories are required by normal body processes like respiration and digestion.

144. A: To minimize digestive upset, food consumed close in time to competition should be in small amounts, and high-fat or high-fiber foods (such as choices B and C) are best avoided.

145. A: Performing body mass measurements in the morning without the influence of external factors like food or drink provides a reliable condition because it is the most easily replicated. The two other conditions could have more variable results due to water weight lost in sweat or weight gained from consuming beverages.

146. B: The preparatory period of periodization is when athletes should be building a base level of conditioning to prepare for more intense and/or more specialized movements later in the cycle. Once this base is established, the intensity can start to be varied and ramped up. Increasing intensity while decreasing volume is a goal of the competitive period rather than the preparatory period.

147. B: The general principles of exercise order dictate that exercises should be ordered to allow an athlete to exert maximal force and demonstrate proper technique. Power exercises, such as any variation on the Olympic lifts (snatch, clean, press, jerk), are the most taxing because they require the most skill. Working large muscle groups with multi-joint movements should occur next in the order and then smaller, single-joint movements.

148. A: Torque can be conceptualized as a product of force and the length of the moment arm. The other choices describe two other principles involved in movement—power is the time rate of doing work, and work is the product of muscle force and displacement.

149. C: Overtraining can occur when an athlete's program exceeds the athlete's ability to recover and puts their body systems under excess stress. Overtraining can occur when frequency, volume, and/or intensity are excessive or when rest and recovery are insufficient. Progressing a program through using a different modality is unlikely to cause overtraining on its own.

150. A: A cooldown with active recovery like walking and light stretching allows an increased heart rate to gradually return to normal. The other two options are incorrect, as practice attempts are important for familiarity with test procedures, and non-fatiguing tests should be done first in the testing order.

151. B: Because the star excursion balance test assesses one leg at a time for balance and stability, it could assess differences between legs and therefore could gauge an athlete's post-injury performance for this situation.

152. C: Performing 3–5 attempts allows an adequate number of trials for an athlete to find their 1-RM while minimizing fatigue that could result from doing more attempts.

153. A: The typical recommendation for resistance training is to exhale during the concentric portion of the exercise, which is where the sticking point occurs. The sticking point at a log press would occur as the athlete presses it upward, so the exhale would reinforce a rigid torso and upright spine for the athlete to ideally pass through the sticking point and successfully press the log.

154. B: ATP's breakdown to ADP and phosphate fuels the pulling action, or power stroke, of the myosin crossbridges as they pull on actin filaments. Calcium is not broken down in this scenario but rather is released from the sarcoplasmic reticulum as an earlier step in the sliding filament theory. Endomysium is the connective tissue surrounding each muscle fiber, so it is not something that gets broken down during muscle contraction.

155. C: Reducing the rest period for a resistance training program focusing on muscular endurance would be a logical progression in continuing to overload the muscles to work at submaximal levels;

however, reducing the rest period for a strength or power goal would likely compromise the success of the movements, since these goals require heavier loads.

156. C: IZOF, or Individual Zones of Optimal Functioning, notes that individuals have individualized levels of arousal. The same stimulus or emotion can affect two individuals in very different ways.

157. A: Muscles function by pulling on bones (never pushing), while tendons are the attachments joining muscles to bones, enabling this movement.

158. A: The principal action in an emergency is to provide immediate care to the affected person. This may require first aid, CPR, or AED, so it is critical that strength and conditioning professionals obtain and maintain current certification, so they are ready to respond immediately in event of emergency.

159. B: While the main muscle fiber types, types I and II, are genetically determined, the subtypes can change with training. For example, type IIx can become type IIa; however, the main muscle fiber types are unlikely to significantly change with training—for example, an athlete with mostly type I fibers is unlikely to shift them to type II fibers even with extensive training.

160. B: While the fibroblastic repair phase still warrants careful consideration for the injured area as it is the second phase of three, relative rest is a general goal of the first phase (inflammatory response phase). Once the injured tissue has passed the inflammatory response phase, it can sustain some function and movement and should not need to be isolated with rest.

161. B: Placing a mirror at least 20 inches above the floor gives a 2-inch buffer to prevent weight plates from damaging or breaking the mirror since standard weight plates are 18 inches wide.

162. C: Failing to vary training and include adequate recovery places more stress on the adrenal system, causing it to release cortisol. Cortisol by itself is not a negative hormone, but having chronic levels in the body in response to excess stress would be undesirable for training adaptations.

163. B: Velocity can be conceptualized as speed with direction. Speed describes only how fast an object is moving, but velocity incorporates the direction. Acceleration would involve changes in an object's velocity, and agility would involve the capacity to change direction while decelerating and re-accelerating.

164. A: In a superset, two exercises are performed that target opposing muscle groups or areas. The muscles of the chest and shoulders are an antagonist to the muscles of the back and vice versa. Choices B and C target the same general muscle groups in both exercises.

165. B: Using a countermovement, such as swinging the arms back for jumping over a barrier or performing a standing long jump, allows the athlete to work at higher velocity and thus to jump higher or farther. Many plyometric drills use a countermovement, but the lateral push-off does not—it simply starts with the athlete standing laterally to a box with the close foot atop the box, then pushing through that foot to jump up.

166. C: Self-controlled practice is a tactic that can enhance motivation through involving athletes in decision-making (such as providing choices) and promoting their active involvement.

167. C: Making specific nutrition recommendations is out of the strength and conditioning professional's scope, unless they also have specific nutrition credentials, such as a registered dietician (RD). While MyPlate is a useful general resource, athletes who are excluding food groups—such as those eating a vegan diet, which excludes all animal-based products like meat, dairy, and eggs—are highly recommended to work with a sports dietitian so that nutrient requirements for performance can be adequately met.

168. B: A test can be reliable (having high consistency or repeatability) without being valid (measuring what it is supposed to measure). In this case, a 12-minute run test could be easily done as a repeated measurement and likely get consistent results, meaning high reliability; however, this test selection is not a valid application for measuring strength, as the 12-minute run measures aerobic capacity.

169. B: Interval training is stressful on the body, as it involves training at high intensities close to VO_2 max. Thus, keeping the rest equal to the work portion is beneficial. The other two choices have significantly more work than rest in their ratios.

170. B: Supercompensation is described as part of the general adaptation syndrome, a model explaining how the body responds to stress. When the body is overloaded with a stressor that is not excessive and is well structured, the body compensates with improved performance.

171. C: A mission statement should address the target clientele, what service is being provided, and what makes the service unique. While hours and location are important, that information is neither part of conveying why the organization is distinctive nor what it contributes.

172. B: The practice technique of simplification means that the task difficulty is adjusted. Here, a back squat is easier to perform with a light barbell, allowing the athlete to gain practice in proper technique without the task being too difficult.

173. C: Maintaining a forward trunk lean and keeping the head in line with the spine during the acceleration phase of a sprint helps the athlete to maximize acceleration. Otherwise, bringing the head or torso into a more upright, lifted position can detract from the body's ability to accelerate.

174. C: Stressing the phosphagen system to provoke the most ideal training adaptations would involve near-maximal intensities and adequate recovery to prevent overtraining and foster energy system and muscular adaptations. Regarding the other choices, intensity and duration have an inverse relationship (high intensities cannot be performed for long durations), and lower intensities would not be the most accurate means to stress the phosphagen system.

175. A: The drive phase of using a rowing machine is when the athlete begins to pull with the arms, pushing through the legs as the hips and knees extend.

176. C: Out of the listed choices, a power goal would have low repetitions (such as 1–5, depending on type of event) and multiple sets (3–5). While this volume is appropriate for power, the number of reps is too low for a hypertrophy goal or an endurance goal.

177. A: State anxiety is characterized by an individual's subjective perception of feeling apprehensive or uncertain about a situation, which is typically accompanied by arousal that is not well controlled, leading to symptoms of anxiety like a racing heart.

178. A: Based on the sport-specific needs of soccer, aerobic endurance is a foundational quality. Such foundational capacities should be built well before the preseason or the in-season so that the athlete has the proper base for more specialized movements or qualities needed to prepare for competition.

179. C: Content validity refers to the extent to which a test, or battery of tests, covers appropriate component abilities. Since gymnastics requires power, strength, and flexibility, the choice of tests should be valid for assessing the specific needs of the sport.

180. A: The pathway of inspired air in the respiratory system (after air is inhaled through the nose or mouth) is to the trachea, then to the bronchi of each lung, then to the smaller bronchioles, and lastly to the alveoli. The capillaries are a site of exchanging oxygen but are not a direct part of the respiratory system's path during inspiration.

181. C: Traffic flow is a critical aspect in building and designing a new facility, as understanding the number of athletes who will be using the facility at any given time ensures that everyone can have safe and easy access.

182. B: Vitamin C is a water-soluble vitamin that also serves as an antioxidant. Colorful fruits and vegetables, including oranges, peppers, tomatoes, and others, are all high in vitamin C.

183. A: High GI (glycemic index) foods are more quickly digested and absorbed than lower GI foods. White bread is considered a high GI food, with a ranking of 70+.

184. B: The role of the strength and conditioning professional is not to diagnose or to treat an eating disorder or a suspected eating disorder, as this is out of the scope of the role, which rules out choices A and C; however, it is the strength and conditioning professional's responsibility to help the athlete receive proper care and diagnosis through referral to a qualified professional.

185. A: Targeted rehabilitation for an injured athlete would be in the scope of a sports medicine professional. A strength and conditioning professional's scope includes working with athletes who have injuries and working to prevent injuries from happening, but specific rehabilitation post-injury would be beyond the scope of practice for the role.

186. A: Synergists indirectly assist in movement, such as stabilizing structures so that the prime movers, or agonists, can contract and the antagonists can decelerate the movement and provide additional stability.

187. B: The Valsalva maneuver is best used for structural exercises that load the spine, such as a back squat, as it can help promote a rigid, neutral spine through alignment and support.

188. B: Systolic blood pressure increases with exercise because it represents the work of the heart's ventricles to eject blood. Diastolic pressure will slightly decrease (due to vasodilation) or stay the same.

189. A: Muscle dysmorphia is an altered self-perception where an individual feels the need to increase their body size and muscle mass based on feeling overly small and weak—sometimes resorting to high-risk measures like steroid use.

190. B: The Krebs cycle and the electron transport system are incorrect choices because they are aerobic, occurring in the mitochondria and requiring oxygen.

191. A: The cross-sectional area of a muscle fiber enlarges primarily due to increased myofibrils, which then increase the size of the overall muscle. The other choices are possible training adaptations, depending on the stimulus, but are not directly linked with muscle hypertrophy.

192. A: The barbell back squat can be performed with a variety of foot positions. This may mean a narrow, medium, or wide stance. The toes should be pointed slightly out, up to 30 degrees from neutral; the exact angle should be that which is most comfortable for the athlete. No matter what the foot placement, the heels should be firmly planted on the floor throughout the exercise.

193. B: In the front squat, the barbell is held in front of the body, where either the parallel-arm position or the crossed-arm position can be used for placement of the bar on top of the anterior deltoids.

194. B: Inter-rater reliability refers to the consistency in different raters' agreement on results over time. In this situation, because one coach is not utilizing the same standardized protocol, the results are likely to be more inconsistent.

195. A: Viewing an athlete from the frontal plane will best allow assessment of the knees being positioned over the toes rather than going inward (i.e., valgus knees). Ensuring proper alignment is critical for safe landing in plyometrics and preventing injury.

196. A: Knowledge of performance feedback allows an athlete to understand their movement patterns, which could be done through videos or other equipment.

197. A: Primary needs of basketball include strength, power, and agility. Of the listed choices, the standing long jump and the star excursion balance test are less directly specific to the needs of the sport than the T-test, as selecting the test is the main key in discerning the right answer. While theoretically any of the resistance training movements could have a case for being used in a basketball player's program, the hang clean and push press go toward maximizing power and jumping needs.

198. B: Underwater weighing and DEXA are "gold standard" methods that assess amounts of lean mass and fat mass. Skinfolds, when assessed correctly, are more accurate than circumferences as they measure subcutaneous fat and not just girth.

199. B: Heart rate reserve is the difference between an athlete's maximal heart rate, measured in a laboratory during exercise testing, and resting heart rate. Because this process requires an athlete to undergo laboratory testing procedures to assess their actual maximal heart rate, this will allow the strength and conditioning coach to assign the training intensities for the athlete more accurately. This is superior to age-predicted methods and the Karvonen method for estimating aerobic training intensities.

200. C: An unloading week is intended to reduce overall training stress on the athlete before engaging in the next phase of the training period. This is generally intended to allow the athlete to recuperate sufficiently and begin to express some, if not all, of the trained capacities of the prior phase. This concept serves as a means for one phase to build on top of another and to avoid overreaching in the short term and overtraining in the long term. An unloading week can be very useful for athletes moving from a hypertrophy phase with significant volumes to a combination strength/hypertrophy phase with higher loading and increased training volumes or from a strength phase heading into a competition period.

201. A: The Yo-Yo intermittent recovery test is characterized by short bursts of work in shuttle runs with short recovery periods. This test is preferable to a steady-state aerobic test to mimic the demands of team sports that have frequent starts and stops.

202. C: The demands of volleyball include explosive lower body power, like that which is required in jumping. A plyometric program for volleyball would thus include various types of jumps relevant to the needs of the sport. For safe and effective jumping, proper landing technique is essential, and since most jumps land in a squat variation, using the squat would allow assessment of the athlete's form.

203. B: Combination training is a type of cross-training that requires an anaerobic athlete to train aerobically for a period to facilitate recovery from prior training sessions. There is some debate as to the overall effectiveness of this approach when considering the traits and characteristics of an anaerobic athlete's sport, as training aerobically may cause a reduction in muscle size, strength, and power.

204. A: An upper/lower split training approach will allow the athlete to gain the necessary lean mass in the upper torso, hamstring, and quadriceps because each session will have significantly higher volumes than if the athlete were to train using a total body approach. This body part split will also allow the athlete to use big compound movements, both structural and power movements, without interfering with the recovery of other muscle groups that may be involved in these exercises, as would be the case with a whole-body approach.

205. B: For the most valid and reliable results out of the three listed tests, non-fatiguing tests should go first, of which skinfolds or other body composition measurements are an example. Agility tests should go next because they are high skill and could be impacted by fatigue from other tests, like a 1-RM test. Out of the choices here, the 1-RM bench press would then be the last, as the two tests before are unlikely to significantly affect it.

206. A: Volume and intensity will generally receive the most focus across a periodized plan; however, volume and intensity can each be manipulated in various ways, such as the load lifted or the total distance run, for example.

207. B: A SWOT analysis (Strengths, Weaknesses, Opportunities, and Threats) should occur in the second half of the predesign phase. This is an important step before any type of design or construction to ensure the facility will be most successful.

208. B: In the steps of a needs analysis, once the evaluation of the sport's needs has occurred, the strength and conditioning specialist needs to evaluate the athletes on training status through physical testing and evaluation. This will help determine the program's goal. These lacrosse players may be very untrained in resistance training or may be highly advanced athletes. Performing a step like selecting exercises or using power exercises is jumping too far ahead. The strength and conditioning specialist must first understand the training status of the athletes.

209. B: The Karvonen method first takes the age-predicted maximum heart rate ($220 - \text{age}$, which in this case is $220 - 43 = 177$). Next, subtract the individual's resting heart rate from the resulting number (which in this case is $177 - 53 = 124$). This number is then multiplied by each end of the range, and the resting heart rate is added back in to each range calculation. The results can be rounded to the nearest whole number:

$$(124 \times 0.65) + 53 = 133.6$$

$$(124 \times 0.75) + 53 = 146$$

210. A: A basketball player who is shooting a free throw must use the primary movers for the upper body, which include the triceps, the pectoral muscles, the deltoids, and the biceps, along with the forearm flexors and extensors. Using an overhead pressing movement for strength development in a basketball player meets the specific needs of the athlete's sport by targeting and training the specific muscle groups involved in this action.

211. C: Variable practice means that variations of the same skill are performed in a single session. Here, the skill is the quick feet lateral agility drill, but the different equipment provides novel variations on the skill.

212. C: The first attempt for a 1-RM should be approximately 50% of the estimated 1-RM weight. In this case, 50% of 220 lb (100 kg) is 110 lb (50 kg).

213. C: Cardiac output is the product of stroke volume and heart rate. Thus, if an athlete has a greater stroke volume, this will cause the end product (cardiac output) to increase.

214. A: The lactate threshold is the exercise intensity where blood lactate begins to abruptly increase and the need for anaerobic energy production also increases. Trained individuals can perform at higher intensities before the lactate threshold is reached.

215. B: Osteoblasts respond to mechanical loading of the bone, such as in resistance training, through laying down collagen that stimulates new bone formation, making the bone stronger.

216. B: The athlete's position on the volleyball court dictates that she will need sufficient strength and muscular resiliency in her pressing musculature as well as in her upper back. To meet this requirement, she will need to train at sufficient loading intensities to develop the strength in the targeted upper body musculature, and this can effectively be achieved with 70–85% loading intensity. At this intensity level, she will develop over the entire off-season program. To develop muscular resiliency and work capacity, she will need to train with a sufficient number of repetitions per set, which should fall between 6 and 10 repetitions.

217. C: When setting resistance training goals, the most important factor is ensuring that the final resistance training goal is attainable in the current sport season. In the example provided, the desire to add 10 lb (4 kg) to the deadlift, from 405 lb to 415 lb (184 kg to 188 kg), is a reasonable goal in the eight-week off-season training period. This goal will not require the athlete to engage in any special behaviors or to access substances or specialized training methods to obtain it.

218. C: For safe and effective exercise progression, a general guideline is not to increase the frequency, intensity, or duration by more than 10% each week. Based on the athlete's current amount, they are running 120 minutes per week. Option C adds on 12 total minutes (10% of 120) with the two slightly longer runs. Option A decreases the running amount, which does not go toward progression, and option B increases both the days per week and the running amount for a total of 175 minutes, which is far above a 10% increase.

219. C: Using a superset approach during the in-season training program increases the amount of work performed in a brief window of time. During the in-season training period, time is at a premium due to other obligations that include practice, film study, position and team meetings, etc. Using a superset approach will allow the athlete to train with great focus and intensity for a brief period, and this will benefit the athlete during the season by maintaining strength, stamina, and other work capacities that may decrease during the season.

220. A: Volume-load is a way to quantify the work performed in resistance training and involves multiplying the total sets by the reps in each set and the weight lifted per rep. This problem can be solved by working backward. If 2,580 lb (1,170 kg) is the end result, this can be divided by the sets (4), then the reps (3), resulting in the correct weight lifted. This number can be re-checked for accuracy by multiplying 4 sets by 3 reps and the chosen weight.

CSCS Practice Test #2

1. Caffeine is a heavily studied ergogenic aid and has a myriad of positive effects on performance. Which of the effects listed below is NOT one of them?

a. Increased fat oxidation
b. Enhanced memory
c. Increased neuromuscular feedback

2. When transitioning to a preseason training period, what modifications will the strength and conditioning coach make to the training parameters for the athletes?

a. Increase training load intensity.
b. Decrease training load intensity.
c. Increase training volume.

3. What are the primary goals for the strength and conditioning program, either as a private company or a university athletic department?

a. Individual development through a team setting
b. Decreasing potential injury risks and improving performance
c. Developing athletes mentally and physically

4. During a pro-agility test, what must occur for the attempt to count?

a. The athlete's hand must touch the cone.
b. The athlete's foot must touch each line.
c. The athlete must run past each line.

5. Foods such as cake, cookies, and ice cream can be categorized as:

a. Low in nutrient density
b. Low in caloric density
c. High in nutrient density

6. In the off-season training program, how often should the athlete resistance train?

a. 4–6 training sessions per week
b. 1 training session per week
c. 2–3 training sessions per week

7. A 200-meter hurdler is about to begin his competitive training season. What training approach would the strength and conditioning coach use to maintain the athlete's explosive and work capacities?

a. Complex training
b. Circuit training
c. Compound sets

8. What protein is responsible for initiating muscular contraction?

a. Myosin
b. Tropomyosin
c. Troponin

9. An athlete needs to develop specific movement patterns to gain mastery in his sport. What is the guiding principle for this type of training, and what skill type needs to be trained?

a. Skill specificity; closed movement skill
b. Practice specificity; closed movement skill
c. Skill specificity; open movement skill

10. What type of foods would be most optimal for an athlete to consume during and immediately after exercise?

a. Foods that are high in dietary fiber
b. Foods that are high in omega-3 and omega-6 fatty acids
c. Foods that are high-GI (glycemic index)

11. What connective tissue attaches a muscle to a bone?

a. Ligament
b. Cartilage
c. Tendon

12. When adjusting a cam-, pulley-, or lever-based exercise machine, what is the most important consideration for the athlete's body position?

a. Making sure the athlete is aligned with the angle of push or pull
b. Ensuring the primary joint involved in an exercise is aligned with the axis of resistance
c. Discussing optimal body position and demonstrating proper movement execution

13. When evaluating the body fat composition of high school-aged female athletes using a skinfold measurement procedure, what sites are tested?

a. Thigh, subscapular
b. Suprailiac, biceps
c. Suprailiac, triceps

14. A strength and conditioning professional wants to assess aerobic capacity in soccer players. Which of the following tests would be best suited for this purpose?

a. Margaria-Kalamen test
b. Yo-Yo intermittent recovery test
c. 300-yard shuttle

15. Which of the following is an example of content validity in an athlete testing scenario?

a. A group of gymnastics athletes is assessed with a battery of multiple tests, with each test relevant to an aspect of their sport.
b. An aerobic capacity test is found to correlate directly with athlete performance on a cross-country team.
c. An overhead squat test is used to represent necessary requirements for stability and mobility in novice Olympic weightlifters.

16. What muscle fiber type has the greatest capacity for force production and hypertrophy?

a. Type IIa
b. Type IIf
c. Type IIb

17. Which of the following symptoms would be most likely to indicate anorexia nervosa?

a. Osteopenia
b. Increased red blood cell count
c. Bronchospasm

18. What is an impulse with regard to speed and agility training, and how is this measured?

a. A shift in momentum as a result of force, (Impulse = Force × Time)
b. A shift in momentum as a result of force, (Impulse = Force/Time)
c. The rate of directional change as a result of force, (Impulse = Force × Time)

19. What is the primary limitation of trunk plyometrics?

a. Limited stretch-reflex response
b. Too many muscle groups involved
c. Hip flexors overtaking the abdominals

20. When a client is performing a bench press, where should the trainer's hands be placed to spot the client effectively?

a. Center of the barbell using an alternated grip
b. Center of the barbell using a pronated grip
c. Outside the athlete's hands in a pronated grip

21. During the repair phase, what is the primary objective of treatment?

a. Prevent muscle atrophy and joint deterioration
b. Maintain joint mobility and increase muscular elasticity
c. Prevent disruption of tissue healing

22. Why is backpedal running considered to be a specific and independent movement pattern and not simply the reverse of forward sprinting?

a. Different force couplings at the hip and thigh
b. Anatomical and functional asymmetry of the leg
c. Alternate muscle firing patterns

23. Which of the following movements are open-chain movements?

I. Bench press
II. Lunge
III. Leg curl
IV. Lying triceps exercise

a. I and III only
b. I, II, and IV only
c. I, III, and IV only

24. Which of the responsibilities below is NOT within the purview of the strength and conditioning coach?

a. Develop and implement training programs.
b. Assess injuries.
c. Provide skill and movement corrections during training.

25. Which of the body positions below is NOT a necessary part of correct positioning for a bench press?

a. Buttocks are firmly and evenly placed on bench
b. Shoulders and upper back are on bench
c. Lower back is arched to increase spinal stability

26. In the off-season program for a Premier League soccer player, training volume and intensity are characterized by what during the strength/power phase?

a. High intensity and low volume
b. Low intensity and high volume
c. Low intensity and low volume

27. Which anatomical plane splits the body into left and right segments?

a. Frontal plane
b. Transverse plane
c. Sagittal plane

28. Under what physiological conditions will gluconeogenesis take place?

a. Periods of starvation
b. Excess carbohydrate consumption
c. Periods of protein deprivation

29. A strength and conditioning professional plans to do skinfold measurements on an athlete as part of a test battery. Which of the following is necessary for the most reliable results?

a. Skinfolds should be done after anaerobic or power testing since they are non-fatiguing.
b. Skinfolds should be taken in the morning with the athlete in a fasted state.
c. Skinfolds should be done before any type of exercise.

30. Out of the following, what element of training is most important for effective agility technique?

a. Maximizing ground contact time
b. Eccentric muscular contractions
c. Utilizing unilateral movements

31. A high school football coach decides to bench the starting running back after a fumble early in the first half. The coach's decision is an example of what type of reinforcement?

a. Positive punishment
b. Negative reinforcement
c. Negative punishment

32. Which of the following is a common error with arm movement in sprinting technique?

a. Arms move into the transverse plane
b. Elbows drive down and back
c. Hands break at the waist

33. Under what conditions would using high-GI foods prove most beneficial to an anaerobic power athlete?

a. After a restorative flexibility training session
b. After a high-intensity and low-volume resistance training session
c. After a high-intensity and high-volume resistance training session

34. When designing training programs for children, what area of adaptation to resistance training is a concern?

a. Skeletal adaptations
b. Neuromuscular adaptations
c. Cardiovascular adaptations

35. How many vertebrae are in the cervical region?

a. 5
b. 7
c. 12

36. When preparing for a training session or athletic event, what type of stretching should be avoided?

a. Dynamic stretching
b. Ballistic stretching
c. Static stretching

37. What is a benefit of using variable practice?

a. It allows for more complex skills to be broken down into smaller parts, promoting mastery.
b. It promotes being responsive and flexible in responding to novel and unpredictable environments.
c. It allows an athlete to get real-time feedback on their technique and performance and adjust accordingly.

38. Which of the options below is representative of steps an athlete should take to return to normal training processes during the remodeling phase after an injury?

a. Isotonic strengthening to dynamic stretching
b. Concentric strength to eccentric strength
c. Flexibility to eccentric strength

39. A track and field coach is designing a training program for a broad jumper. In what order should the selected exercises be performed in this program?

I. Power clean
II. Hamstring curl
III. Reverse hyperextension
IV. Deadlift

a. IV, I, III, II
b. I, IV, III, II
c. IV, III, I, II

40. What energy system is most active during brief, intense muscular contractions?

a. Anaerobic glycolysis
b. Phosphagen system
c. Gluconeogenesis

41. Which athlete in the following scenarios is most likely to be experiencing bulimia nervosa?

a. A rowing athlete always makes excuses not to eat with the team after practices and weighs themselves multiple times a day.
b. An ice-skating athlete has a body mass index of 20 and tracks their macronutrient percentages at each meal.
c. A track athlete frequently consumes multiple servings of desserts in secret, followed by running many extra miles outside of practice.

42. What causes metabolic acidosis?

a. Rapid decrease in enzyme activity, resulting in increased lactate accumulation
b. Rapid increase of hydrogen ion concentration in the blood that causes a decrease in blood pH
c. Rapid increase in enzyme activity, resulting in decreased lactate accumulation

43. Which of the following contributors to total energy expenditure can an athlete most easily change?

a. Basal metabolic rate (BMR)
b. Physical activity
c. Diet-induced thermogenesis

44. When designing a plyometric training program for younger athletes, what should the focus of the program be?

a. Increased power
b. Skill acquisition and movement-specific strength
c. Skill acquisition and neuromuscular control

45. Inactivity and poor nutritional habits lead to the downregulation of this hormone, resulting in significant disease complications over time. What is the hormone?

a. Oxytocin
b. Insulin
c. Cortisol

46. A high jump athlete experienced a badly sprained ankle during a run-up for a jump while in competition. They have recovered from their injury and are clear to begin training high jump again, but have developed a fear of jumping because they do not want to get injured again. Which of the following strategies best demonstrates using counterconditioning with this athlete?

a. Helping the athlete make changes in their run-up technique to minimize the past association with the injury
b. Creating a pre-jump routine that involves a series of contracting and relaxing muscles head to toe
c. Guiding the athlete through visualizing each step of their run-up while emphasizing relaxation through breathing

47. If a marathon runner uses a four- to six-week training block to swim and cycle, this is considered to be what kind of training?

a. Alternative training
b. General endurance training
c. Cross-training

48. When training for strength and power, which adaptations will occur most quickly?

a. Neural
b. Muscular
c. Cardiovascular

49. What is the correct starting position for the feet in performing the snatch?

a. Just inside hip-width or shoulder-width with the feet pointing forward
b. Hip-width or shoulder-width apart with toes pointed slightly out
c. In a wide sumo stance with the feet and knees pointing out at about a 45° angle

50. When evaluating athlete readiness for engaging in a plyometric program, what are the primary considerations?

a. Balance, strength, flexibility, speed
b. Balance, technique, flexibility, strength
c. Strength, technique, balance, speed

51. What phase of an ECG represents ventricular depolarization?

a. P-wave
b. QRS complex
c. Q-wave

52. Which substance is responsible for supplying the energy for human movement?

a. Glycogen
b. Acetylcholine
c. Adenosine triphosphate

53. Addressing a muscular weakness, primarily as a contributor to a compound movement, would require the inclusion of what kind of movements?

a. Assistance
b. Isolation
c. Structural

54. A cross-country runner wants to improve their lactate threshold. Which training technique would be most effective?

a. Tempo training
b. Long, slow distance training
c. Bodyweight circuit training

55. Tapering is an important component of competition preparation. What is NOT a primary benefit to a tapering strategy before competition?

a. Neurological recovery
b. Joint/muscle recovery
c. Increased glycogen stores

56. During the second transition phase, a collegiate baseball player should engage in which of the following activities?

a. Free swimming
b. High-intensity interval training
c. Motocross

57. What is the difference between oxygen debt and oxygen deficit?

a. Oxygen deficit refers to the initial anaerobic energy system contributions, and oxygen debt is the volume of oxygen consumed above resting values.
b. Oxygen deficit is the volume of oxygen consumed above resting values, and oxygen debt refers to the initial anaerobic energy system contributions.
c. Oxygen deficit is the volume of oxygen consumed during rest before exercise, and oxygen debt refers to the difference between the volumes of oxygen consumed between resting and exercise values.

58. What is the recommended amount of floor space for the stretching area per athlete?

a. 49 square feet
b. 58 square feet
c. 40 square feet

59. If training an athlete to improve work capacity or a specific characteristic such as speed endurance, what type of resistance training split and method could be used to enhance the anaerobic conditioning activities the athlete would necessarily undertake?

a. Total body training
b. Circuit training
c. Upper/lower split

60. What training adaptation to aerobic exercise increases the end-diastolic volume?

a. Right ventricular hypertrophy
b. Left ventricular hypertrophy
c. Left atrium hypertrophy

61. If a strength and conditioning coach wants to improve sprint speed, what type of lower body plyometric drills would be most effective over a six-week plyometric program?

a. Jumps in place; box jumps for height
b. Single-leg jumps in place; single-leg jumps for height
c. Horizontal bounding; single-leg jumps

62. Which of the following plyometric drills would have the highest intensity?

a. Depth jump with lateral movement
b. Alternate-leg push-off
c. Backward skip

63. What component of a program is most important when specifically training to improve speed endurance?

a. Training frequency
b. Exercise relief patterns
c. Training volume

64. A member of the strength and conditioning facility is wearing blue jeans to train in the facility. What are the proper actions for a strength and conditioning coach or associate staff member to take for this first-time rule violation?

I. Verbal warning by a staff member
II. Dismissal from the facility for the day
III. Make the member aware of the violated rule
IV. Document the offense

a. I and II
b. I and III
c. I, III, and IV only

65. A volleyball athlete is evaluated on the sit-and-reach, vertical jump, T-test, and power clean. The athlete's lowest percentile scoring is in the T-test. What should their training focus on to improve their scores for the future?

a. Agility drills, such as changing direction in response to a stimulus
b. Straight line speed, such as effective technique for acceleration
c. Anaerobic power, such as explosive exercises

66. An athlete struggling with physical manifestations that affect athletic performance positively or negatively is an example of what type of anxiety?

a. Somatic anxiety
b. Physical anxiety
c. Perception anxiety

67. Out of all of the needs of an athlete, the sport needs of the athlete are most important. Which athlete listed below would benefit most from a moderate-volume, moderate-intensity training program in the off-season?

a. Swimmer
b. Discus thrower
c. Football player

68. What is the translation point for the muscular and nervous systems?

a. Neuromuscular junction
b. Peduncle
c. Motor neuron

69. Why are capillaries significant for optimal function in the vascular system?

a. They transport large volumes of oxygenated blood to working tissues.
b. They transport hormones, exchange fluids, gases, and electrolytes with interstitial fluids throughout the body.
c. They exchange large volumes of CO_2 and O_2 with the lungs.

70. The feasibility study establishes what essential element for the strength and conditioning facility?

a. Determines facility demographics
b. Outlines services to be provided
c. Establishes total cost

71. When programming power and structural movements in the same session, what repetition ranges and training intensities will the strength and conditioning coach most likely assign?

a. Power: 1–5 repetitions at 70–80%; Structural: 8–10 repetitions at 80–90%
b. Power: 3–5 repetitions at 75–85%; Structural: 4–6 repetitions at 80–90%
c. Power: 3–8 repetitions at 85–90%; Structural: 10–12 repetitions at 75–85%

72. Which of the following is the correct order of exercises for warming up an athlete for competition?

I. Sport skill
II. Dynamic stretching
III. Jogging
IV. Bounding

a. III, I, II, IV
b. IV, II, I, III
c. III, II, I, IV

73. What cardiovascular rhythm is indicated by a resting heart rate of less than 60 beats per minute?

a. Tachycardia
b. Atrial flutter
c. Bradycardia

74. A strength and conditioning professional is testing a group of Senior Olympians (50+ years of age) who will be competing in the 50 m and 100 m run at their next event in a few months. The professional wants to use a 40-m straight-line sprint test to assess the athletes; however, there is no normative data for this demographic to use for comparison. The best option in this case is:

a. Use the normative data that exists, even if it is not for the same demographic.
b. Select a different test that does have normative data for 50+ year olds, such as the 12-minute run.
c. Use the athletes' own results for comparison, such as scores before and after 2 months of training.

75. When assessing a basketball player's one-legged jumping ability, the strength and conditioning coach notices the athlete does not jump very well off his left leg. What movement pattern and training strategy would the coach select to begin the process of correcting this issue?

a. Include instability training using unstable surfaces.
b. Include unilateral lower body movements.
c. Include additional bilateral lower body movements.

76. A triple jumper is completing training preparations for the World Championships in four weeks. What phase of preparation is the triple jumper in at this point in the training program?

a. Competition; transition preparation
b. Competition; end preparation
c. Competition; peaking

77. When an athlete is lifting maximal or near-maximal loads throughout a training cycle, what is the most effective method for maintaining progress and balancing training stress?

a. Varied training volume
b. Varied training load intensity
c. Block training

78. What are the key elements of a pre-competition meal that ensure maximum benefit to the athlete?

a. Meal timing, well-tolerated food choices, meal macronutrient content, enjoyable food selection
b. Meal macronutrient content, low salt, proper carb and protein balance, enjoyable food selection
c. Meal timing, proper hydration procedures, high protein content

79. Hormone responses to resistance training play a key role in muscle hypertrophy. Which resistance training program design will maximize the response of testosterone and growth hormone?

a. High volume, light load, and short rest periods
b. Low volume, heavy load, and long rest periods
c. High volume, heavy load, and short rest periods

80. The preparatory phase is the longest training phase in a yearly macrocycle. What is the primary emphasis for this training phase?

a. Initiation of higher training volumes
b. Establishment of a baseline of conditioning
c. Preparation for higher-intensity loading

81. Which of the athletes listed below would benefit most from a circuit training approach?

a. In-season basketball player
b. Marathon runner
c. Deconditioned football player

82. Which situation requires multiple spotters to assist an athlete should they miss a lift?

a. An athlete performing a maximum repetitions test at 225 lb (102 kg)
b. An athlete squatting 450 lb (204 kg) in a work set
c. An athlete overhead pressing 185 lb (84 kg)

83. Which of the following situations describes actions that are outside of the scope of practice for the strength and conditioning professional in the context of mental and psychological health?

a. An athlete is concerned about their levels of anxiety before competition. The strength and conditioning professional helps the athlete understand and implement some basic stress management techniques.
b. A strength and conditioning professional notices that an athlete has seemed quiet and withdrawn during the last few training sessions. The strength and conditioning professional starts a conversation with the athlete asking about aspects like their sleep, energy, and motivation to gauge if the athlete needs further support.
c. A strength and conditioning professional encounters an athlete purging by vomiting in the gym bathroom after a team lunch. The strength and conditioning professional offers to confidentially help the athlete with their bulimia.

84. During altitude training, there are several acute training adaptations. What are they?

I. Increased pulmonary ventilation
II. Increased myoglobin concentrations
III. Increased capillary density

a. I
b. I and II
c. II and III

85. What is the primary role of an athletic trainer in regard to injuries?

a. Assigning training protocols to injured athletes
b. Management and rehabilitation of injuries
c. Discussing injuries with the strength and conditioning coach

86. How can the strength and conditioning coach structure a training session to account for when an athlete is not performing at or near their normal capacities?

a. Use goal repetitions.
b. Increase rest periods.
c. Reduce training loads.

87. 1-RM testing for power exercises, such as the push jerk, hang power clean, or power snatch requires:

a. A spotter for safety and injury prevention
b. An Olympic-style barbell and safe area to drop the bar
c. A force plate for accurate power measurement

88. When training an athlete with a weakness in a small muscle group, what type of movement will the strength coach prescribe?

a. Auxiliary movement
b. Assistance movement
c. Isolation movement

89. When performing power cleans, the bar is caught in what position?

a. Full squat
b. Half squat
c. Quarter squat

90. Which of the bone injuries listed below occurs most frequently?

a. Stress fracture
b. Displaced fracture
c. Comminuted fracture

91. Which of the following is the recommended method for measuring the grip width for the snatch?

a. Measuring ¼ inch outside of the snatch rings on the barbell
b. Measuring elbow-to-elbow
c. Measuring wrist-to-elbow

92. A female Olympic weightlifter has had her body composition assessed through skinfold measurements, resulting in a percent body fat calculation. Which of the following percentages would be most typical for this athlete?

a. 12% body fat
b. 23% body fat
c. 35% body fat

93. How does ketosis adversely affect an aerobic endurance athlete?

a. Increased substrate circulating in the blood
b. Decreased physical endurance
c. Decreased body fat

94. Which of the following athletes is most likely to be susceptible to a potential dietary iron deficiency?

a. A 19-year-old female soccer athlete
b. A 28-year-old male shot-put athlete
c. A 62-year-old female tennis athlete

95. Which of the following would be the best way to increase stored glycogen in the days leading up to a competition or athletic event?

a. Limit carbohydrate consumption to foods that are primarily low-GI (glycemic index).
b. Consume 8–10 grams of carbohydrates per kilogram of body weight.
c. Restrict carbohydrates during the day, then eat a carbohydrate-rich meal in the evening.

96. Which static stretch would be most effective for an athlete who complains of tight hamstrings?

a. Supine knee flex
b. Forward lunge
c. Butterfly stretch

97. Before each competition, a wrestling athlete experiences feelings of apprehension and dread, along with tense muscles and extreme difficulty focusing. Which mental health condition is most likely associated with the athlete's symptoms?

a. Dissociative disorder
b. Depressive disorder
c. Anxiety disorder

98. An athlete is performing the side quadriceps stretch after a workout. What joint actions need to occur for this stretch to be most effective?

a. Knee flexion and lumbar extension
b. Knee flexion and hip extension
c. Knee flexion and thoracic extension

99. There are several changes in cardiovascular function due to chronic aerobic training. Which of the responses below is NOT one of these adaptations?

a. Increased resting heart rate
b. Increased cardiac output
c. Increased stroke volume

100. What structure is found in both the conduction and respiratory zones of respiration?

a. Primary bronchi
b. Alveoli
c. Bronchioles

101. Which exercises would be selected to generate the highest release of human growth hormone?

I. Compound movements affecting large muscle groups
II. Isolation movements affecting individual muscle groups
III. Loading intensity > 80% and higher training volume
IV. Loading intensity < 70% and lower training volume

a. I and III
b. II and III
c. I and IV

102. Which of the following exercises below represents a first-class lever?

a. Biceps curl
b. Dumbbell lateral raise
c. Triceps extension

103. A strength and conditioning professional is preparing a warm-up for athletes to do the pro-agility test. What movements are most appropriate as part of the warm-up?

a. Partner PNF hamstring stretch, heel to toe walk, front plank
b. Forward lunge with elbow to instep, walking knee lifts, low-intensity side shuffles
c. Arm swings, partial curl-up, spinal twist

104. Which enzyme is responsible for catalyzing the cross-bridging action in muscular contraction?

a. ATPase
b. Calcium ATPase
c. Myosin ATPase

105. What is the purpose of an ECG test?

a. An ECG is used for determining the blood pressure of an athlete post-training.
b. An ECG is used to record the rhythm of the heart, assess blood pressure, and generate information regarding the position and size of the patient's heart.
c. An ECG is used to assess the electrical signals generated during polarization and depolarization of cardiac tissue, which provides insight into the overall function and health of an athlete's heart.

106. Which type of skill would best be learned with whole practice rather than part practice?

a. A basketball layup
b. A vertical jump
c. An Olympic lift

107. Every year at the start of the new season in high school football, the head coach pairs each member of the varsity team up with a younger, less experienced junior varsity member. The junior varsity team members watch the varsity team members go through basic agility drills before it is their turn. Which source of building self-efficacy does this situation best describe?

a. Vicarious experience
b. Performance accomplishments
c. Imaginal experience

108. What percentage of the 1-RM would facilitate developing an athlete's ability to accelerate and increase speed?

a. 50–60%
b. 40–50%
c. 60–70%

109. When wanting to bring up a lagging body part either to overcome a muscular weakness or increase muscular size, what approach could the strength and conditioning coach insert into the training program for a 4–6-week period?

a. Complex training
b. Compound set
c. Circuit training

110. When designing a training program, a strength and conditioning coach uses both structural movements and core movements. How are these movements similar and different?

a. Both affect multiple joints and large muscle groups, but core movements require higher force outputs because they are speed and power movements.
b. Both affect multiple joints and muscle groups, but structural movements load the spine either directly or indirectly.
c. Both affect large muscle groups, but structural movements are always high-force movements and should be placed first in a training program.

111. Morphology of the neuromuscular junction is affected by anaerobic training in what way?

a. The length of nerve terminal branching is increased, and acetylcholine circulation increases.
b. The surface area and length of nerve terminal branching is increased, and synapse locations are increased and dispersed more widely.
c. The surface area is increased, synapse locations are increased and dispersed more widely, and acetylcholine circulation increases.

112. Which of the following aspects would be most effective to enhance perceptual-cognitive ability in an agility drill?

a. Pairing the drill with a dynamic strength movement
b. Performing the drill at slow speeds that gradually increase
c. Incorporating a decision-making skill, such as a coach command

113. What factor should most heavily influence the type of progression method a strength and conditioning coach uses across the different sport seasons throughout the training program?

a. Controlling training stress
b. Gradual training load increases
c. Reducing injury

114. Which of the following exercises does NOT require a spotter?

a. Barbell row
b. Step-up
c. DB incline press

115. From the list of plyometric drills listed below, determine the correct order from least demanding to most demanding.

I. Jumps over an object
II. Depth jump
III. Box jumps
IV. Vertical jump

a. IV, III, II, I
b. IV, I, III, II
c. IV, III, I, II

116. What does the sarcoplasmic reticulum store that is significant for muscular contraction?

a. ATP
b. Calcium ions
c. Sodium/potassium

117. What type of substance is most likely to be misused by an athlete experiencing muscle dysmorphia?

a. Methamphetamines
b. Anabolic steroids
c. Beta-2 agonists

118. Which of the following tests would be potentially contraindicated for an individual with hypertension?

a. Body composition assessment using skinfold calipers
b. Muscular strength assessment using 1-RM back squat
c. Flexibility assessment using overhead squat

119. Utilizing heavy resistance exercises and movements that utilize the stretch-shortening cycle is considered what type of training?

a. Complex training
b. Combination training
c. Contrast training

120. Which of the terms listed below represents an area of legal concern that can be mitigated by a clearly defined emergency care plan for a new strength and conditioning facility?

a. Tort
b. Negligence
c. Eligibility criteria

121. A strength and conditioning professional is instructing a group of athletes on performing a PNF partner stretch for the hamstrings. For the most effective stretch, the athlete who is being stretched should:

a. Contract the quadriceps during the passive phase of the stretch.
b. Hold their breath during the passive phase of the stretch.
c. Alternate between contracting and relaxing their hamstring muscles during the passive phase of the stretch.

122. A basketball athlete is tested on their 1-RM back squat, bench pull, and power clean. The athlete scores in the 85th percentile for the back squat and bench pull and in the 50th percentile for the power clean. Which of the following statements is most likely true?

a. The athlete needs to improve their technique in high-speed strength movements.
b. The athlete needs to improve their levels of low-speed strength.
c. The athlete needs to improve their levels of local muscular endurance.

123. Which of the following is a main recommendation for athletes in strength and power sports?

a. Consume protein after resistance training workouts.
b. Consume an omega-3 supplement regularly to promote muscle recovery
c. Consume foods high in vitamin C to reduce inflammation

124. At what phase of linear sprinting is the stretch-shortening cycle used the most?

a. At deceleration
b. At acceleration
c. At maximal velocity

125. When designing a resistance training program for a rugby player, what should NOT be part of a coach's assessment?

a. Training status
b. Movement analysis
c. Comparative strength analysis

126. Which neuromuscular structure is responsible for initiating the stretch reflex?

a. Muscle spindle
b. Golgi tendon organ
c. Pacinian corpuscle

127. What percentage of the one-repetition maximum will generally allow an athlete to complete eight repetitions per work set?

a. 87%
b. 93%
c. 82%

128. Counterconditioning is a combination of two techniques that are utilized to overcome performance anxiety. What are these two techniques?

I. Hypnosis techniques
II. Reciprocal inhibition
III. Cognitive techniques
IV. Somatic techniques

a. I and II
b. II and III
c. III and IV

129. A strength and conditioning coach is using a sequenced training model. What should the next training block emphasize if an athlete has just completed a block that emphasizes agility?

a. Strength
b. Speed
c. Power

130. When outlining professional responsibilities in the strength and conditioning facility, what position is responsible for supervising the training sessions for the athletes?

a. Athletic trainer
b. Head coach of the athlete's sport
c. Assistant strength and conditioning coach

131. Under what conditions is using the Valsalva maneuver appropriate?

I. In experienced and properly resistance-trained athletes
II. Under maximal loading during structural exercise
III. Under heavy loading during assistance exercises
IV. When performing heavy-resistance abdominal exercises

a. I and IV
b. II and III
c. I and II

132. A basketball athlete does a drill that requires them to shoot the ball from multiple spots on the court, such as a layup and a three-point shot, while guarded by a defender. This is an example of:

a. Repetitive-part training
b. Variable practice
c. Simplification

133. When would using a body part training split be appropriate for an athlete in an off-season training program?

a. To correct muscular imbalance
b. To increase muscle size
c. To recover from an injury

134. What other disorders frequently co-occur in individuals with eating disorders?

a. Depressive disorder and anxiety disorder
b. Avoidant personality disorder and obsessive-compulsive disorder
c. Bipolar disorder and dissociative disorders

135. What is the name of the outermost layer of muscle fiber?

a. Epimysium
b. Endomysium
c. Perimysium

136. When determining what equipment to purchase for a new strength and conditioning facility, this decision should be most heavily influenced by which person?

a. Strength and conditioning director
b. Director of business operations
c. Facility manager

137. During muscular contraction, two specific proteins form a crossbridge that generates movement. What are these two proteins called, and for what actions during the crossbridge formation are they individually responsible?

a. Actin is the thin filament and serves as the binding site. Myosin is the thicker filament and forms the crosslink to the actin filament.
b. Troponin is the thin filament and serves as the binding site. Tropomyosin is the thicker filament and forms the crosslink to the troponin filament.
c. Myosin is the thick filament that serves as the binding site during muscular contraction. Actin is the thin filament that serves as the crosslink during muscular contraction.

138. Which fiber type is most important to an endurance athlete?

a. Type IIa
b. Type I
c. Type IIb

139. A baseball player takes two practice swings before stepping into the batter's box before each at bat during a game. What is this athlete demonstrating?

a. Preparatory routine
b. Procedural routine
c. Performance routine

140. Which pair of muscles has an antagonistic relationship?

a. Biceps and latissimus dorsi
b. Rectus abdominis and erector spinae
c. Gastrocnemius and soleus

141. During the starting position of the snatch, what coaching cue should be given to an athlete who starts with his chest over the barbell and hips higher than the shoulders?

I. Squat down with the hips lower than the shoulders
II. Eyes focused straight ahead or slightly downward
III. Shoulders over or slightly in front of the bar
IV. Chest held up and out

a. I, II, and III
b. II and III
c. I, III, and IV

142. What type of training should be recommended to an aerobic athlete who wants to improve his anaerobic metabolism but is concerned about overtraining?

a. High-intensity interval training
b. Steady state training
c. Fartlek training

143. What energy system supplies the majority of ATP when the body is at rest?

a. Aerobic glycolysis
b. Phosphagen system
c. Oxidative system

144. When assigning training volumes during periods of maximal or near-maximal lifting intensities, a coach must consider what specific element when completing a program outline?

a. Increasing total training volumes for the week
b. Current strength levels of the athletes
c. Need for increased recovery time

145. When training an athlete who needs to perform multiple explosive events in a short period of time, what intensity and repetition range should a strength coach prescribe?

a. 80–90% intensity for 1–2 repetitions per set
b. 75–85% intensity for 3–5 repetitions per set
c. 67–85% intensity for 3–5 repetitions per set

146. Which testing procedure would be the best for assessing an athlete 's speed?

a. 400-meter sprint
b. 150-meter sprint
c. Pro-agility test

147. After performing the essential assessments of an athlete's strength, balance, and speed, what is the next step in the assessment process?

a. Perform a vertical jump test to establish a vertical jump baseline.
b. Assess movement and flexibility of the athlete.
c. Evaluate the athlete's jumping technique.

148. Which of the following is a primary duty and responsibility of a strength and conditioning professional?

a. Provide initial care in response to an emergency.
b. Create informed consent forms to reduce the risk of negligence claims.
c. Provide clearance for an athlete to participate after recovering from an injury.

149. A basketball player stands at the free throw line, focused on the rim, and is preparing to shoot the first of two free throw attempts. He effectively ignores the raucous noise of the home crowd and makes both attempts. What ability is this athlete using?

a. Selective focus
b. Selective attention
c. Discriminating focus

150. What are the primary functions of hemoglobin?

I. O_2 transport
II. CO_2 transport
III. Acid base buffer
IV. Deliver nutrients to muscles

a. II and IV
b. I, II, and III
c. I and III

151. Which of the training phases below is an alteration to the Matveyev model of periodization?

a. Competition phase
b. Strength/power phase
c. Transition phase

152. Which muscle fiber type has the greatest capacity for morphological and physiological adaptations in response to long-term aerobic training?

a. Type IIb
b. Type IIx
c. Type I

153. During warm-ups, a lacrosse player notices that his right hamstring is a bit tighter than normal, so he spends an extra five minutes of the warm-up period performing light static and dynamic stretching. He plays and presents with little to no evidence of having any remaining hamstring stiffness. The athlete has taken advantage of what muscle quality?

a. Tension
b. Elasticity
c. Plasticity

154. Other than adding additional training load for an athlete, what other mechanisms that utilize the progressive overload principle are acceptable for athlete progression?

I. Increasing repetitions performed at specific loading parameters
II. Increasing work density
III. Increasing number of sets performed at specific loading parameters
IV. Reducing rest periods

a. I, II, III, IV
b. I and III
c. I, II, and III

155. What is the most important element to consider when determining the training frequency for an athlete?

a. Sport season
b. Training status
c. Exercise selection

156. When an athlete drops from the top of a box and first contacts the ground, what are the phases of the stretch-shortening cycle after ground contact has occurred?

a. Reactive, transition, concentric
b. Reactive, amortization, rebound
c. Eccentric, amortization, concentric

157. Of the following substances, which is NOT considered an ergogenic aid?

a. Protein powder
b. BCAAs
c. Acetaminophen

158. What anatomical structure is considered to be the "pacemaker" of the heart?

a. Sinoatrial node
b. Bundle of His
c. Atrioventricular node

159. When designing a training program, a strength coach includes a box jump for maximum height in a superset with front squats. What neurological phenomenon is the coach attempting to utilize?

a. Stretch-shortening cycle
b. Myotatic stretch reflex
c. Potentiation

160. In the modified Matveyev model, in which phase do sport-specific activities begin?

a. Hypertrophy/endurance phase
b. Basic strength phase
c. Peaking phase

161. What is the muscle structure responsible for controlling muscular responses to rapid changes in muscle tension to prevent injury?

a. Golgi tendon organ
b. Muscle spindle
c. Lamellar corpuscle

162. Which of the following supplements would be most likely to have adverse effects if used by an athlete?

a. Branched-chain amino acids
b. Caffeine-containing energy drinks
c. Anabolic steroids

163. If equipment limitations are an issue at a training facility, what test could be used most effectively for determining maximum muscular power?

a. Margaria-Kalamen test
b. Vertical jump
c. Pro-agility test

164. What is the prescribed push-up testing standard from the American College of Sports Medicine?

a. As many repetitions as possible in 2 minutes, resting at the peak when necessary
b. As many repetitions as possible in 60 seconds
c. As many repetitions as possible, performed continuously, until failure

165. Rest periods are extremely important for allowing muscular and neural recovery between sets. What is the suggested rest period between sets for an athlete with a goal of muscular endurance performing 4 sets of 12 repetitions in the squat?

a. 2–5 minutes
b. 1–2 minutes
c. 20 seconds

166. What role, if any, does strength play in determining an athlete's maximal sprint velocity?

a. Strength allows an athlete to overcome increased resistance generated on the body as acceleration occurs.
b. Strength is what propels an athlete forward when attempting to accelerate the body.
c. Strength is essential for the initial takeoff to propel the body forward and sustain the sprint effort.

167. When determining the effectiveness of a training program, when should the strength and conditioning coach perform a final review?

a. End of the in-season program
b. End of the competition year
c. End of the off-season program

168. A male cross-country athlete was assessed on the 1.5-mile run, resulting in an estimate of their VO_2 max. Which of the following values would indicate a very high level of aerobic capacity?

a. A VO_2 max of 42 mL/kg/min
b. A VO_2 max of 54 mL/kg/min
c. A VO_2 max of 66 mL/kg/min

169. For many years, daily protein intake for athletes has been recommended at levels similar to the recommendations for non-athlete populations. What is the current recommendation?

a. 0.8–1.3 g/kg of body weight
b. 1.9–2.3 g/kg of body weight
c. 1.4–1.8 g/kg of body weight

170. Which substance is heavily involved in muscle anabolism and neurological adaptations?

a. IGF
b. Cortisol
c. Testosterone

171. When working with an athlete with limited training experience, what is the most appropriate way to assess strength levels?

a. 15–20 repetition maximum
b. 6–8 repetition maximum
c. 10–12 repetition maximum

172. What cue would be most effective for the position of the spine during the descent portion of the squat?

a. "Lift the chest."
b. "Extend the hips."
c. "Arch the lower back."

173. What is made up of long, thin chains of proteins that are arranged into sarcomeres and responsible for muscular contraction?

a. Myofilaments
b. Actin
c. Myofibrils

174. The first step in designing a training program is to undertake what two-step task?

a. Injury analysis
b. Needs analysis
c. Physiological analysis

175. The sarcolemma in striated muscle tissue plays a significant role in muscular contraction. What is the primary function of the sarcolemma?

a. The primary function of the sarcolemma is to conduct electrical signals via the neuromuscular junction.
b. The primary function of the sarcolemma is to conduct electrical signals via transduction, signaling the release of Ca^{2+} ions.
c. The primary function of the sarcolemma is to pump Ca^{2+} ions into and out of a muscle cell.

176. During the inflammatory phase of injury recovery, what kind of training can be undertaken by the athlete?

a. Maintaining strength and endurance in adjacent muscles
b. Isometric contraction of injured area
c. Lightly stretching the injured area

177. When performing a data analysis on the effectiveness of the strength and conditioning program for three similar female sports—volleyball, basketball, and sprinting and jumping—what statistical approach to the data should the strength and conditioning director use?

a. Central tendency
b. Difference score
c. Variability

178. What periodization model would be most effective for an athlete who has multiple events during a competitive season?

a. Linear periodization
b. Non-linear periodization
c. Matveyev periodization

179. The protein hormone erythropoietin (EPO) can be used to enhance aerobic endurance. Via what mechanism does EPO improve aerobic function?

a. Increased plasma volume
b. Increased renin-angiotensin-aldosterone activity
c. Increased hematocrit

180. Which valves of the heart are responsible for preventing backflow into the ventricles during diastole?

a. Semilunar valves
b. Tricuspid valve
c. Atrioventricular valves

181. Members of a volleyball team are undergoing a test battery at the beginning of their season. Which of the following test sequences would be most effective and reliable?

a. 1-RM power clean, vertical jump, and pro-agility test
b. Pro-agility test, 1-RM power clean, and vertical jump
c. Vertical jump, pro-agility test, and 1-RM power clean

182. Which of the listed training volumes will affect muscular hypertrophy the most?

a. 5 sets of 10 repetitions
b. 5 sets of 5 repetitions
c. 3 sets of 8 repetitions

183. How will increased activity in the parasympathetic nervous system (PNS) affect athletic performance?

a. Increased activity in the PNS will affect athletic performance positively via increased focus and mental acuity while also enhancing neural signaling for muscular contraction.
b. Increased activity in the PNS will affect athletic performance negatively, as this system is responsible for a reduction in mental focus and body temperature and is most active during leisure activities.
c. Increased activity in the PNS will affect athletic performance positively via increased activity of the cardiorespiratory and endocrine systems.

184. When determining the methods to include in a sprint training program, where do sprinting, sprint assistance, mobility, and endurance training fall in order of importance?

I. Sprinting
II. Endurance training
III. Sprint assistance
IV. Mobility

a. I, II, III, IV
b. I, IV, III, II
c. I, III, IV, II

185. Which testing procedure represents the best layout for a test battery?

I. 1-RM squat
II. Pro-agility
III. Pull-up test
IV. 110-meter sprint test

a. II, I, IV, III
b. II, III, I, IV
c. III, I, IV, II

186. In Olympic lifts like the clean and the snatch, when does extension of the hips, knees, and ankles occur?

a. During the first pull
b. During the second pull
c. During the catch

187. If a 100-meter sprinter has a problem with pulling their hamstring frequently, what would be a prescription for their in an off-season program to help eliminate this issue?

a. Increase conditioning work.
b. Increase training frequency.
c. Improve strength ratios at the affected joints.

188. A strength and conditioning professional is working with a new group of high school athletes. The strength and conditioning professional has the athletes sign an informed consent form but is eager to get them working out and does not get assessments of their medical histories. Which term describes the potential consequences if one of the athletes gets injured?

a. Negligence
b. Violating scope of practice
c. Assumption of risk

189. Which of the following is the most effective form of PNF (proprioceptive neuromuscular facilitation) stretching?

a. Hold-relax with agonist contraction
b. Hold-relax
c. Contract-relax

190. What is the primary issue with this spotting technique in the dumbbell bench press?

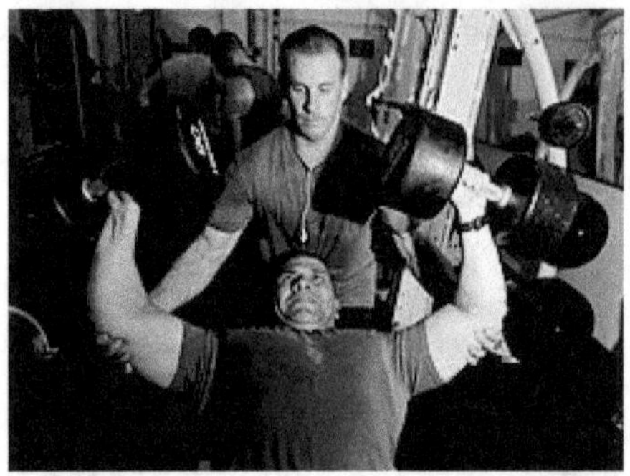

Licensed Under CC BY-SA 3.0 (creativecommons.org/licenses/by-sa/3.0/)
https://commons.wikimedia.org/wiki/File:US_Navy_101122-N-7948R-111_Chief_Warrant_Officer_Jose_Martinez_performs_dumbbell_chest_presses_in_the_gymnasium_aboard_the_amphibious_dock_landing.jpg

a. The spotter should not be touching the athlete.
b. The athlete should not be spotted at all for safety concerns.
c. The spotter should be spotting at the athlete's wrists.

191. A RAMP protocol is being used to create a warm-up for a soccer athlete. The first activities are ones that elevate the heart rate, such as short shuttle runs and side shuffles, and the warm-up continues with lunging and rotating patterns. What type of activity would come next for an effective RAMP warm-up?

a. Sport-specific soccer agility drills
b. Dynamic stretches
c. Longer-distance running

192. What is one of the primary adaptations to energy production due to chronic aerobic exercise?

a. Increased mitochondria density in muscle tissue
b. Increased oxygen-carrying capacity of hemoglobin
c. Increased glycogen storage capacity

193. A baseball athlete confides in the assistant coach that one of their teammates has been misusing amphetamines to improve their performance. What sign or symptom would indicate amphetamine use in the athlete?

a. Loss of balance and coordination
b. Erratic and restless behavior
c. Aggressive and hostile demeanor

194. What equipment is needed to accurately administer the YMCA bench press test?

a. A tape measure to determine the athlete's grip width
b. A contact mat system to measure the amount of contact time
c. A metronome to provide audible signals

195. How is pyruvate utilized if not enough oxygen is available during glycolysis?

a. Pyruvate is converted via fermentation to lactate to produce sufficient ATP.
b. Pyruvate is converted to acetaldehyde to produce sufficient ATP.
c. Pyruvate is converted to acetyl coenzyme A, then to alanine, and then to ATP.

196. A group of cycle athletes is doing high-intensity interval training (HIIT) for aerobic conditioning. Which work-to-rest ratio would be most appropriate to use?

a. 1:20
b. 1:12
c. 1:1

197. A coach wants to use guided discovery for an athlete learning the deadlift. Which of the following would be the most accurate example of this?

a. The coach tells the athlete to lift the bar off the floor while keeping a flat back.
b. The coach guides the athlete to feel that both feet are evenly pressing into the floor.
c. The coach has the athlete do the deadlift at a slower pace using an empty bar.

198. Cartilaginous and synovial joints differ in what specific aspect?

a. Cartilaginous joints do not allow significant movement, and synovial joints allow significant movement.
b. Cartilaginous joints comprise ligaments and tendons but lack the synovial fluid compartments that are found in synovial joints.
c. Cartilaginous joints are tough, fibrous, uniaxial joints, and synovial joints are capsulated, multiaxial joints.

199. A gymnast is learning a balance beam routine, which includes a roundoff, then back handspring, and then a back tuck. The coach directs the gymnast to practice multiple roundoff repetitions, multiple back handspring repetitions, and then multiple back tuck repetitions before trying all three movements in succession as part of the routine. This best describes:

a. Pure-part training
b. Random practice
c. Explicit instructions

200. During a combine event, there are 12 separate timers during the 40-yard dash event. What is the best approach for accurately collecting and reporting the data?

a. Remove the highest and lowest times and then assess the average.
b. Calculate the average of all 12 timers.
c. Determine the standard deviation among the times.

201. Which of the following is accurate regarding the testing procedure for the standing long jump and vertical jump tests?

a. Ground contact time is measured as part of the athlete's score.
b. Doing a countermovement will invalidate the score.
c. The score is the best of three trials.

202. What initiates the upward phase of a kettlebell swing?

a. Spinal extension
b. Shoulder flexion
c. Hip and knee extension

203. After establishing baseline testing values, what is the key element for accurately tracking changes over time?

a. Testing frequently (e.g., at least once per week)
b. Testing at regular intervals
c. Testing in similar conditions

204. A marathon runner is preparing to compete in a race located in a hot, desert climate. What should they prioritize most for optimal nutritional performance during their race?

a. Eating small amounts of higher-fat foods during the race
b. Consuming a sports drink with electrolytes
c. Minimizing fluid intake

205. An athlete is trying to reduce their intake of saturated fats. Which of the following should they minimize or avoid?

a. Corn oil
b. Soybean oil
c. Palm oil

206. Which of the following athletes is most likely to experience dehydration?

a. A wrestling athlete using diuretics to lose weight
b. A football athlete using creatine to improve muscular strength
c. A track and field athlete using beta-alanine to improve high-intensity performance

207. Which of the following is best avoided during stretching?

a. Activation of the muscle spindle
b. Creating autogenic inhibition
c. Stimulating the Golgi tendon organ

208. What is the correct position for the shoulders in the starting position for the snatch and the clean?

a. Slightly behind the bar
b. Over or slightly in front of the bar
c. Slightly in front of the hips

209. Which of the following would be the best example of intrinsic feedback?

a. An athlete doing front squats is cued by their coach to keep their eyes forward as they lift.
b. An athlete uses an app on their phone to record the weight they have lifted for their back squat.
c. An athlete uses a mirror to check their knee alignment during a single-leg squat.

210. What is the primary factor for achieving maximal sprint velocities?

a. Stride length
b. Length of recovery phase
c. Stride frequency

211. Using the Valsalva maneuver is helpful when transitioning from eccentric to concentric lifting phases. What is the name for this transition?

a. Sticking point
b. Turnaround point
c. Isokinetic point

212. Which of the following injuries is NOT an overuse injury?

a. Stress fracture
b. Contusion
c. Tendinitis

213. Which scenario is the best example of part practice?

a. A swimmer works on their technique by practicing their arm stroke separately from their leg stroke.
b. A football athlete does sprints repeatedly to improve their speed on the field during games.
c. A weightlifting athlete does extra mobility techniques for their hips and shoulders prior to their training session.

214. In performing the snatch, which of the following would be a technique error?

a. The feet leave the ground in the second pull.
b. The athlete performs the catch with flexion at the knees.
c. The hips rise before the shoulders in the first pull.

215. Which of the following would be most appropriate in the Activate and Mobilize phase of the RAMP Protocol?

a. Cardiovascular activities, such as moderate-intensity jogging
b. Dynamic stretches, such as inchworms or spiderman crawls
c. Higher-intensity preparatory movements, such as speed drills or agility drills

216. An athlete seeking to gain an edge on their performance decides to use a hormone that will increase the amount of oxygen their blood can carry. This best describes:

a. Use of human growth hormone
b. Blood doping
c. 'Stacking' of anabolic steroids

217. How far from lifting equipment should weight trees be placed?

a. 42 inches
b. 36 inches
c. 54 inches

218. Who will the strength and conditioning coach have direct and most frequent contact with on the sports medicine team?

a. Team physician
b. Nutritionist
c. Sports physical therapist

219. Which would be the best aspect of technique to emphasize for achieving a rapid stride rate in sprinting?

a. Maintaining upright posture
b. Full range of motion arm swings
c. Brief ground contact times

220. Which of the following athletes is most likely to have a substance use disorder?

a. A volleyball athlete regularly drinks a mix of branched-chain amino acids and creatine with the goal of building more muscle.
b. An injured weightlifting athlete has started consuming alcohol each night to cope with being unable to train.
c. A track athlete experiences headaches and fatigue after trying to cut down from consuming two energy drinks daily.

Answer Key and Explanations for Test #2

1. B: Caffeine is heavily studied and has been shown to increase fat mobilization in aerobic athletes, increase power output in anaerobically trained athletes, and enhance mental acuity and focus. Caffeine has not been shown to enhance memory or fine motor skills, as caffeine tends to excite the nervous system in a significant way that negatively affects fine motor skills and limits the capacity to focus on a singular task necessary to store subject material in long-term memory for usage on an exam or general recollection purposes.

2. A: In the preseason training phase, the primary consideration for the training program is to increase training intensity while shifting to more sport-specific movements and beginning to focus on technique. Training volumes will also decrease in this phase to allow the athlete to put more energy into sport- and practice-related activities and not negatively affect recovery rates. This change will also reduce the risk of injury heading into the period when the athlete is preparing most heavily for the competitive season, which is about six to eight weeks away when the preseason is initiated. Note that both volume and intensity will vary on a daily, microcycle, and mesocycle basis.

3. B: The primary focus of the strength and conditioning facility is to decrease potential injury risks and to improve athletic performance. The facility may offer a range of services, from restorative massages to blending smoothies, the objective of which is to decrease the risk of injury and improve performance.

4. B: During the pro-agility test, the athlete's foot must touch each line for the testing procedure to count. The athlete makes three separate changes in direction after a brief sprint. When attempting to run quickly, the athlete may stop short of the line, which means the strength and conditioning coach must be very attentive to the athlete's feet touching each line to qualify the time.

5. A: Nutrient-dense foods are those that provide higher amounts of vitamins, minerals, and fiber, such as complex carbohydrates like vegetables and whole grains. Cake, cookies, and ice cream are not typically high in vitamins, minerals, and fiber, so they would be considered low in nutrient density.

6. A: During the off-season training program, an athlete should be training as frequently as possible, with four sessions per week being the bare minimum. More experienced athletes should train more frequently to stimulate progress, as training frequency is one of the key elements for athlete development in a resistance training program as the athlete matures in training age and experience. The other aspect in consideration is the lack of other activities to distract from the training program, as there are no sport-specific activities the athlete is engaging in, and recovery from session to session can be maximized because energy is solely directed to the training program.

7. A: An athlete who requires a high work capacity coupled with the ability to be explosive for brief periods of time will benefit most from using a complex training approach, as this will allow the athlete to use low-moderate plyometric activity during the in-season program to maintain explosive capacities and resistance train at sufficient levels to maintain strength. This type of training does not need to be high-intensity to be effective and can allow an athlete to sustain a high level of performance throughout a training season as long as the strength and conditioning coach closely monitors training volume and intensity.

8. C: Troponin is the protein responsible for initiating muscular contraction, as this is the location where actin and myosin sites bind, forming the crossbridges necessary for contraction to occur. Calcium ions are responsible for initiating the movement of troponin from the myosin binding site, initiating a conformational change. Once this takes place, the myosin crossbridge can be carried out, and muscular contraction can occur.

9. B: Athletic development for sports requires that general and specific tasks be performed to develop coordination, retain movement patterns, and transfer skills to the sport, along with the sensorimotor elements needed to perform in the athletic environment, which falls under the overarching principle of practice specificity. The athlete in the example needs to develop closed movement skills to enhance technique and execution of the required skills for his sport.

10. C: Foods that are high-GI (glycemic index) are digested and absorbed quickly. Some examples include bread, rice, potatoes, and cereal. Eating these during and/or immediately after exercise can provide and maintain energy stores of glycogen. Foods high in fiber or fat are not recommended during exercise because they take longer to digest and may cause gastrointestinal distress.

11. C: A tendon is a fibrous connective tissue made primarily of collagen that connects muscle to bone via the bone periosteum. The tendon bridges the muscle and bone together, facilitating movement throughout the body. Ligaments are also dense fibrous connective tissue that connect bone to bone to hold a joint together. Cartilage is a flexible connective tissue found in numerous joints, including the knee, elbow, and rib cage. Cartilage is more rigid than muscle tissue and absorbs force well, but it is less rigid than bone.

12. B: The athlete must be in proper alignment for the desired joint to be loaded correctly with utmost safety and for optimal movement execution. To achieve this when using a machine or pulley system, a seat, ankle, arm, chest, or back pad may need to be adjusted.

13. C: When testing body composition in high school-aged female athletes, measurements must be taken at the suprailiac and triceps sites. For high school-aged male athletes, the testing procedure calls for the measurements to be taken at the thigh and subscapular sites. These sites allow for consistent measurement and fall in line with where young men and women from an athletic population will typically store fat.

14. B: The Yo-Yo intermittent recovery test assesses aerobic capacity through a shuttle run between two markers 20 meters apart with 10 seconds of recovery. The runs increase in speed through auditory signals, and the athlete continues if they can maintain the increasing pace. The Margaria-Kalamen test measures maximum muscular power (high-speed strength) with a timed staircase run. The 300-yard shuttle measures anaerobic capacity by recording the fastest time to complete six 50-yard sprints.

15. A: Content validity is the extent to which testing covers all relevant abilities or components. Most sports require more than one ability, so administering a battery of tests is common to ensure that no relevant ability is neglected.

16. C: Type IIb fibers are considered "fast" glycolytic, produce large amounts of force, and possess the greatest capacity for hypertrophy. Type IIb fibers primarily function in high-force, explosive-type movements because of the force generation capacities they possess. This fiber has minimal involvement in moderate-duration movements past the initial effort, usually 5–8 seconds, and virtually no impact on sustained muscular contractions and endurance-related efforts.

17. A: Osteopenia is a reduced bone mineral density, making the bones thinner and more brittle. Individuals with anorexia nervosa are more likely to have osteopenia because excessive calorie restriction results in bones not getting adequate nutrients.

18. A: An impulse changes the momentum of an object as a result of a force (Impulse = Force × Time) and is required to achieve a predetermined momentum in less time or greater momentum in a set period. This is why high rates of force production are needed to generate the requisite momentum to move an object, such as an athlete sprinting down the track from a dead start in a set time.

19. A: Trunk plyometrics do not necessarily function the exact same way as upper and lower body plyometrics, and this is due to limited stretch-reflex response. The muscles of the trunk do not effectively store elastic energy, which limits the capacity of the trunk musculature to generate reactive force. Research findings suggest that slow response times and lower movement velocities result from the distance between the trunk musculature and the spinal cord.

20. A: Spotting a barbell bench press by placing the hands at the center of the barbell using an alternated grip ensures that the spotter will not lose grip suddenly if the athlete is struggling to complete a set or has missed a maximum intensity load attempt.

21. A: During the repair phase of tissue healing, the treatment focus is on preventing muscle atrophy and joint deterioration. This phase must be handled delicately, as the newly regenerated tissues, primarily collagen, are still vulnerable to stress, so a low-load stress process must be undertaken while still working to prevent the joint from losing range of motion. This process will allow the joint to stabilize and the tissues to heal sufficiently to begin the next phase of healing, the remodeling phase.

22. B: The distinction between the two patterns arises from the mechanical constraints on the two movements due to the anatomical and functional asymmetry of the leg and is evident in the kinetics and kinematics of each. Backpedal running is characterized by shorter stride length, increased stride frequency, greater support phase time, and smaller range of motion at the knee, hip, and ankle joints.

23. C: Differentiating between open- and closed-chain movements is important when assigning exercises to injured individuals. This is because exercise selection should follow a natural development path as the athlete heals and can produce greater force through a joint. It should begin with an open-chain movement, which can typically be performed on a machine or with dumbbells to allow free joint movement but also control the amount of resistance being used to promote the desired training effect. Closed-chain movements tend to be big compound movements that allow for large forces to be produced using free weights (e.g., squats, lunges, deadlifts, or overhead presses). The key is understanding when to use a closed- or open-chain movement in an injured athlete's programming to provide the greatest benefit.

24. B: The strength and conditioning coach is not involved in the assessment of injuries during either a competition or a training session. The strength and conditioning coach should never provide medical advice, as this is not within his scope of responsibilities or the scope of his training and education. In case of an emergency, the strength and conditioning coach can provide CPR/AED or first-aid support until medical personnel arrives. This is a legal issue, and the delineation of medical responsibilities falls to those licensed to perform such activities by the state of issuance.

25. C: When performing supine resistance exercises such as a bench press, the body should contact the bench or ground at five points. The head should be firmly in place on the bench or back pad, the shoulders and upper back firmly in place and even on the bench or back pad, the buttocks placed evenly on the bench or seat and under the hips, with both feet placed firmly and flatly on the floor. The lower back may be arched during a bench press depending on athlete goals (such as powerlifting), but it is not necessary to perform the exercise correctly.

26. A: The strength/power phase is the final stage in the preparation phase and is characterized by high-intensity, low-volume training activities. Activities that take place in this training phase include high-intensity plyometric activity, sprinting against resistance, and resistance training that includes power/explosive exercises with heavy training loads and low training volumes.

27. C: The sagittal plane passes through the posterior and anterior aspects of the body and divides the body into left and right halves. Examples of movements that occur in the sagittal plane include leg extensions and biceps curls.

28. A: Gluconeogenesis is the process of proteins being broken down and converted into glucose for energy production. This is not a common occurrence and generally will only be seen in periods of starvation, extended periods of time with low to no carbohydrate consumption, and exercise bouts greater than 90 minutes.

29. C: Skinfolds should be done on skin that is clean and dry for the most reliability, so if they are part of a test battery, they would be done before any tests that require physical activity. Skin that is sweaty could affect the tester's ability to accurately pinch the skin, affecting the reliability of the results; however, it is not necessary for an athlete to be fasted for accurate skinfold measurement.

30. B: Eccentric muscular contractions are essential to effective braking, or decelerating, and agility training involves changes of direction where frequent acceleration and deceleration are present.

31. C: Negative punishment is a form of reinforcement that removes something that is highly desirable, in this case playing time, to deter the negative behavior. Negative punishment is the antithesis of positive reinforcement and is a commonly applied method for behavior deterrence.

32. A: Arms that move into the transverse plane during sprinting can reflect inefficient technique or fatigue, which expends extra energy. Instead, the elbows should drive down and back, remaining in the sagittal plane, with the hands breaking at the waist.

33. C: A high-intensity loading session coupled with high volume will require significant resources to facilitate recovery and tissue restoration because glycogen stores will be significantly depleted, and there will be neural and biochemical fatigue. This type of session must be supported with sufficient caloric intake post-training, with most calories being derived from carbohydrates and proteins and a minimal amount of fats.

34. A: During childhood and adolescence, when undertaking resistance training exercises, protecting the diaphysis of the long bones and the growth cartilage is extremely important in preventing injury to these areas by emphasizing skill and technique acquisition over loading intensity. An adult will be able to handle higher training loads without risk to these areas, as these growth areas will cease growing and solidify between 17 and 22 years of age.

35. B: The vertebral column in the human body can have between 32–34 vertebrae. There are 7 cervical vertebrae, 12 thoracic vertebrae, 5 lumbar vertebrae, 5 sacral vertebrae fused into 1 bone, and 3–5 coccygeal vertebrae fused into 1 or 2 bones.

36. B: Ballistic stretching requires an athlete to be moving or producing muscular force/movement and a rhythmic bouncing action at the end position. This is a dangerous practice due to the activation of the stretch reflex generated by the bouncing action at the end position, as this extends the range of motion after each repetition and can result in damage to the connective and soft tissues of the joint and muscle. Activating the stretch reflex during stretching activities negates the purpose of stretching the tissues to facilitate increased range of motion, as the stretch reflex will increase muscular tension in response to the bouncing action.

37. B: Variable practice uses different skill variations rather than repeated practice on a single skill. For example, a football team using variable practice for agility could use a variety of agility tools, such as ladders or cones. In contrast to practicing the same skill repeatedly (termed blocked practice), variable practice promotes more flexibility to changing situations since sports are not predictable.

38. C: Correctly developing the necessary flexibility and strength capacities to return to training and competition is essential during the remodeling phase of injury recovery. The proper procedure for returning an athlete to normal training includes transitioning from an emphasis on flexibility to developing eccentric strength in the affected muscle to ensure the injured muscle's ability to load without creating too much stress in the injured tissues.

39. B: The strength and conditioning coach must first consider the needs of the athlete, and in this case, the athlete is a broad jumper and will rely most heavily on the posterior chain to propel the body forward and to spring into action out and across the ground. The selected movements will develop the posterior chain sufficiently and will facilitate improvements in jumping distance. The proper training order must be from most demanding and complex to the least demanding and complex. The correct order for the selection given is power clean, deadlift, reverse hyperextension, and hamstring curl.

40. B: The phosphagen system relies on the hydrolysis of ATP from local muscle stores and on the breakdown of creatine phosphate. This system is active during bouts of intense, brief exercise, which includes heavy resistance exercises and short, intense sprints. This system is active during all activities at the outset but is active for a short time before other systems become the primary energy resource depending on the duration of exercise.

41. C: The two main characteristics of bulimia nervosa are binge eating and purging. With binge eating, the individual often eats secretively and in significantly greater amounts than normally would be consumed. The subsequent purging can happen through laxatives, diuretics, vomiting, or excessive exercise.

42. B: Metabolic acidosis is a condition that occurs when the body produces too much acid. In athletes, the condition is induced by intense bouts of exercise that causes a rapid decrease in blood pH due to increased H^+ ions in the blood. This response can be indicative of the current training capacities of an athlete or group of athletes but can also be used to determine proper training intensity levels.

43. B: Out of these three components, physical activity is the only one an athlete can change on a day-to-day basis. For example, if an athlete needs to lose weight, they may choose to pair nutritional changes with expending more daily calories through additional physical activity. While basal metabolic rate (BMR) can be altered through gaining fat-free mass, this would occur over a longer, more gradual time period. Diet-induced thermogenesis, or the thermic effect of food, includes energy-expending activities like digesting and absorbing food. An individual cannot easily change the rate of these body processes.

44. C: Considerations for younger athletes include emphasizing fun, the development of proper technical movement patterns, neuromuscular control, and anaerobic skills necessary to participate in athletic endeavors. Younger athletes will require progression from simple movement skills to more complex skills over time, and consideration for development in the areas of power, strength, and other measurable elements will benefit from the time spent developing proper movement skill and technique execution.

45. B: The downregulation of insulin results in the type 2 diabetes. This is due to the resistance of the insulin receptors in the body's tissue to the secretion of insulin from the pancreas. This resistance is caused in large part by elevated, or uncontrolled, blood glucose levels over many years and is generally coupled with significant periods of inactivity.

46. C: Counterconditioning is the underlying principle behind systematic desensitization. In this case, the desired outcome is to replace the athlete's fear of jumping with a relaxation response instead. The other options do not specifically address replacing the fear response with something else, which is an essential part of counterconditioning.

47. C: An endurance athlete engaging in alternate methods from event-specific training is considered cross-training. Cross-training for brief training segments in a competition year can assist with the recovery from injury or with general recovery during intense periods of competition preparation. Breaking up training segments allows the muscles to be trained in various ways and provides relief to joints that may be overexposed to stress from preparation for competition.

48. A: When training for strength and power, the neural adaptations will occur most quickly due to, in large part, the size principle. The nervous system will recruit all motor units to facilitate maximal force generation, from weakest and slowest-firing to strongest and most rapidly-firing. During strength and power training phases, the high-threshold units are depended on heavily to perform the required work but also become more easily recruited due to a lowered recruitment threshold. This change allows for these motor units to be recruited more effectively and with greater speed.

49. B: Proper foot position for the snatch maintains the body's weight over the middle of the feet both at the beginning and the end of the lift. This is done most effectively when the feet begin at hip-width or shoulder-width with the toes pointed slightly out.

50. C: Before initiating a plyometric training program, an athlete must be assessed for sufficient balance, strength, and speed while also possessing an understanding of proper plyometric technique. These are mandatory elements that must be present before initiating a plyometric training program to reduce the risk of injury, as plyometric movements are high-force, high-velocity movements that carry significant risk if performed incorrectly or with athletes who are not adequately prepared to perform these exercises.

51. B: The QRS complex represents ventricular depolarization of the left and right ventricles. This complex is characterized by three separate components (the Q, R, and S waves), but the small Q and S waves may not be present in all ECG tests. Details of ECG lead placement can affect the waveform, even when cardiac function is normal, and the R and S waves may be so brief as to not be recorded. The R wave is much larger in amplitude than the P wave because of the larger mass of the ventricles of the heart in comparison to the atria.

52. C: Adenosine triphosphate (ATP) is the energy source that the human body requires to carry out endergonic reactions (i.e., muscular contraction). ATP is composed of an adenine group, a ribose group, and three molecules of inorganic phosphates.

53. A: Assistance exercises are movements that recruit smaller muscle groups, involve one primary joint, and serve to balance out muscular imbalances. Exercises that fit into this category can be added to a training program without the strength and conditioning coach being concerned with overtraining or adding substantial training volume to an athlete's program, as these movements do not place significant demand on the neural system and do not require significant loading to elicit the desired training effect.

54. A: Tempo training, also called pace training, is done at or slightly above race pace. Exercising at a higher intensity improves the lactate threshold. Long, slow distance would not promote significant lactate threshold adaptations since the intensity is lower, and bodyweight circuit training, even if done at higher intensities, is not as specific for creating adaptations as running techniques would be in the case of this athlete.

55. A: Neurological recovery is not a primary emphasis in tapering methods, as tapering involves planned technique work and gradually reducing the training duration and intensities. The nervous system, due to the repetitive nature of aerobic endurance training, is not taxed as heavily as it is for anaerobic power athletes, and neurological fatigue will not play a significant role in the success or failure of an aerobic athlete's competitive season. Allowing for joint/muscle recovery, rehydrating, and increasing glycogen stores are of greater importance to the aerobic endurance athlete.

56. A: An athlete who has completed his competitive season should engage in some light activity that is not related to his sport skill. This activity should be a low-intensity, non-baseball sport activity, and free swimming meets the core criteria of the second transition phase. The other activities listed are not excellent choices. High-intensity intervals are too demanding and do not fit into the second transition paradigm. Motocross is a dangerous activity for an athlete to engage in during the off-season.

57. A: The oxygen deficit refers to the early initial contributions of the anaerobic energy systems during a bout of exercise until a steady state of oxygen consumption is achieved. Oxygen debt refers to the increased rate of oxygen above resting rates after an intense bout of exercise.

58. A: The suggested square footage allotment for each athlete in the stretching and warm-up area is 49 square feet. This is to allow for dynamic and static stretching exercises. Each athlete should have ample room to move in the space and to eliminate the possibility of injury due to being too close to one another. If partner stretching is an emphasis in the training program, a large stretching and warm-up area is necessary.

59. A: An athlete who is trying to improve their speed endurance or anaerobic training capacity would benefit most from engaging in a total body training routine that requires the athlete to train using big compound movements at every training session, most effectively using a superset model, and training frequently throughout the week. This approach will develop the resiliency needed for competition, and with proper movement and training load selection, explosive power and strength will also increase significantly.

60. B: With regular aerobic exercise, the muscle fibers of the heart become stretched over time. The left ventricle experiences the largest change, which leads to a greater end-diastolic volume. This morphological change increases the volume of blood ejected during exercise, when increased oxygen uptake is essential for the working muscle tissues and athletic performance.

61. C: Developing sprint speed, which is considered a form of horizontal single-leg bounding, can be achieved effectively using a combination of horizontal bounding and single-leg jumps. These exercises can also be included in a sprinting program before sprint technique and speed work.

62. A: Depth jumps are some of the highest-intensity movements in plyometric drills because they require a great amount of overload and resistance to overcome, along with large amounts of stress on the muscles and joints to land properly.

63. B: Properly administering exercise relief patterns during speed endurance training sessions is very important because the work-to-rest ratio needs to be adequate to facilitate proper neurological patterns and to avoid premature fatigue, but it also needs to challenge the athlete's metabolic responses to become fatigue resistant. To achieve proper work-to-rest ratios, the coach should monitor an athlete's technique when he engages in the training activity and track the training volume from session to session.

64. B: The process that should be undertaken when an athlete or member of the strength and conditioning facility violates a rule for the first time requires the staff member to provide a verbal warning to the member and an explanation of the rule. This verbal reprimand should also include a reminder of the disciplinary action that will be taken for a second offense.

65. A: The T-test measures agility, so if the athlete scored lowest in this assessment, their training would benefit from focusing on enhancing this skill. Volleyball requires rapid changes in direction in response to a stimulus (such as blocking the ball or returning the ball). Agility drills could enhance the athlete's ability to execute these in training and competition.

66. A: Somatic anxiety is a form of anxiety that causes physical manifestations the person cannot determine the cause of, such as butterflies in the stomach before a soccer match. Somatic anxiety can have either positive or a negative impact on performance, as this is dependent on the mental capacity of the person experiencing this type of anxiety. Some athletes can perform under high levels of somatic stress, and others are unable to overcome the stress response and will perform poorly.

67. A: Swimming is not considered a power sport, but the athlete will still need to be explosive in the pool at the starting position and will also need significant strength levels to move through the water as quickly as possible. This type of athlete would not need to train near maximal loading intensities and will not require large training volumes to be successful in the sport. The athlete will need moderate training intensity and volumes to develop the strength and resiliency needed to be successful in the sport.

68. A: The neuromuscular junction is the central communication point for the nervous and musculoskeletal systems that lead to muscular contraction. This is the translation point for the nervous system signal (electrical) that is converted into a biochemical reaction and then into movement (mechanical).

69. B: Capillaries are the smallest of the blood vessels and serve as part of the microvasculature. Capillaries are where the blood exchanges fluids, gases, nutrients, hormones, electrolytes, and other substances with the interstitial fluids from various tissues throughout the body.

70. C: The feasibility study is primarily intended to assess the costs of building and establishing the necessary components of a strength and conditioning facility. The feasibility study also serves to assess the conceptual strengths and weaknesses of a facility as a secondary focus to determine its practical viability and to make changes to the initial business plan and concept.

71. B: When considering using both power and structural movements in a training session, training block, or throughout a training program, the key consideration is neurological fatigue. Power movements are extremely demanding on the nervous and metabolic systems due to the technical and ballistic nature of these movements. This means programming the power movements in the program first is paramount. Limiting the athletes to a training intensity that will allow multiple repetitions per set will generate the greatest performance benefit without risking excessive fatigue accumulation in the long term. Programming the structural movements for moderate loading intensities and training volume will cause significant performance increases as well, due to improving technical skill and developing the muscular strength without pushing the boundaries of neural and metabolic recovery.

72. C: Best practice for competition warm-up begins with movements of a general or lower-intensity activity, which may include jogging, skipping, dribbling a basketball, or throwing a football, to prepare the body for the activity that follows. After the general warm-up period, the specific warm-up activities begin. These consist of dynamic stretching activities, moving from single-joint to full-body movement, followed by specific exercises that that mimic the movements of the sporting event. The warm-up should gradually increase in intensity up to jumping and bounding activities to prepare the nervous system for competition but should not be so intense as to induce metabolic or neural fatigue.

73. C: Bradycardia is an arrhythmia consisting of a resting heart rate below 60 beats per minute. A normal heart rate falls between 60 and 100 beats per minute. Tachycardia is when the resting heart rate is over 100 beats per minute.

74. C: If there is no normative data for a given test and demographic, it is recommended to develop norms by using pre-training and post-training results of standardized testing. Comparing to normative values of a different demographic would not yield a reliable comparison, and selecting a 12-minute run would not be an appropriate test for the primarily anaerobic demands of running 50 m or 100 m.

75. B: Addressing a weakness that occurs on one side of the body is most effectively done by training that side of the body. In this example, adding unilateral lower body training volume will be sufficient to help improve the athlete's one-leg jumping ability. This will not create a deficiency in the right side, as both sides will be trained using this approach. Using a unilateral approach does not mean the elimination of bilateral training, as the athlete can continue to train these movement patterns. The strength and conditioning coach may simply add unilateral training to the program or reduce the bilateral training volume to compensate for the added training volume from the unilateral movements.

76. C: When preparing an athlete for a single competitive event, the proper approach is to engage in a peaking strategy that will push the athlete's performance to the highest level possible for a three-week period. The peaking strategy differs from a maintenance approach of moderate intensity and moderate volumes, as this period calls for very high intensity and very low training volumes to maximize the necessary characteristics for competition.

77. B: The purpose of altering training loads and volumes over the course of a training program is to allow for adequate recovery of the muscles and central nervous system to avoid entering an overtrained state. The strength and conditioning coach can avoid overtraining athletes by reducing and rotating training loads of other training sessions after a "heavy" training session (i.e., "light" and "moderate" sessions) to facilitate recovery while sustaining training frequency and volumes. Rotating the loading parameters between light, heavy, and moderate can be done for a variety of training goals and frequencies while also serving as a method for addressing the physical stress of practice or competition.

78. A: The pre-competition meal should occur three to four hours before competition to avoid gastric discomfort. Athletes should consume a meal that contains all three macronutrients, as this will allow for proper energy and blood glucose levels throughout the competition. Endurance athletes will require larger amounts of carbohydrates as a percentage of total calories consumed because of the energy demands of their sports. All pre-competition meals should be suited to the athlete's preferences and individual differences and responses to various food types and meal composition.

79. C: Resistance training causes increases in circulating levels of several hormones, including the anabolic hormones testosterone and growth hormone and the catabolic hormone cortisol. Resistance training targeting a large muscle mass (e.g., deadlifts, squats) using a combination of high volume, heavy load, and short rest periods maximizes this hormonal response. Excessive workouts can, however, lead to a chronic elevation in cortisol, which can lead to a catabolic state with serious negative effects on training and health.

80. B: The primary focus of the preparation phase is to establish a baseline level of conditioning for the athlete, as this will prepare the athlete for upcoming training phases that require higher intensities and higher training volumes. The preparatory phase is highlighted by lower training load intensities, higher training volumes, and no sport-specific or skill training. This phase is strictly intended as a developmental stage for future training phases.

81. C: In this example, the deconditioned football player would benefit the most from circuit training, as this would allow them to perform a high volume of work with minimum rest periods. This contributes to improving muscular endurance and work capacity in the upper and lower body while also enhancing cardiorespiratory fitness. If the athlete is overweight, this approach will also contribute to shedding the excess body fat.

82. B: An athlete performing a squat with 450 lb (204 kg) should utilize multiple spotters to protect against injury if the lift is missed. While a 225-lb (102-kg) maximum-repetition test could require multiple spotters, the loading is not sufficient to command multiple spotters.

83. C: Actions outside of the scope of practice for a strength and conditioning professional include diagnosing health conditions and providing specific therapy or treatment. It is not in the scope of practice to affirm whether the athlete has bulimia or not, nor is it in the scope of practice to provide specific help for eating disorders; however, it is within the scope of practice for a strength and conditioning professional to provide general performance enhancement and to do fact finding through conversation to see if an athlete may need a referral to a different qualified individual.

84. A: The acute adaptations of altitude training are an increase in pulmonary ventilation and cardiac output in both resting and exercising states. Acute adaptations are necessary to stabilize respiration and heart rate due to the decreased partial pressure of oxygen at altitude. Chronic adaptations to altitude training primarily affect cellular function, take place over four to six weeks, and stabilize after this period.

85. B: The primary role of the athletic trainer is to manage and rehabilitate injuries resulting from training, competition, or other physical activity. The athletic trainer can also assign sport-specific exercises intended to prevent injuries and apply prophylactic equipment for practice and competition to prevent injury or provide stability to an injured muscle or joint via bracing or taping.

86. A: Setting goal repetitions for a training session, such as 3–5 repetitions for 3–6 sets, will allow an athlete to train slightly below their maximal capacity without worrying about a poor performance when they are not at peak ability. This approach serves as a form of auto-regulation, as training intensity and volume are modulated based on the athlete's day-to-day capacity instead of strictly adhering to a rigid set and rep scheme that would force the athlete to attempt to work beyond their capacity, leading to poor performance and possibly compromising a training block or program.

87. B: Power exercises with a barbell require an Olympic-style barbell where the sleeve can rotate to accommodate proper technique and high speeds of movement. Power exercises do not require a force plate. These exercises should not be spotted, as doing so is often unsafe. Rather, the athlete should lift in a designated area, like a lifting platform, where the bar can be safely dropped if the athlete misses the lift.

88. C: When addressing structural weaknesses or a size deficiency in smaller muscle groups, using isolation movements will address the weakness directly. A smaller muscle group will need direct training stimulus to improve neural integration and recruitment patterns, and isolation work will allow the athlete to focus on contracting the weak muscle group and developing the ability to contract the muscle group maximally when using compound movements.

89. C: After reaching triple extension and completing the second pull, the athlete pulls the body under the bar and rotates the arms under and around the bar. At this point, the hips and knees are flexed to a quarter squat position. Once the bar reaches the clavicle and is stopped, the athlete stands from the quarter squat position, thus completing the lift. The quarter squat is preferred over the full catch position because of the inherent injury risks of performing such a highly skilled movement pattern with inexperienced athletes.

90. A: Stress fractures are the most common type of fracture among athletes due to the high forces generated repetitively during practices, training sessions, and competition. Stress fractures will also most often occur when training volume suddenly increases or an athlete accumulates significant training stress on hard training or competitive surfaces.

91. B: The preferred methods of assessing the correct grip width for the snatch lift is to measure from elbow-to-elbow or fist-to-opposite shoulder. Either approach is acceptable. Taller or longer-armed lifters benefit from the fist-to-opposite shoulder method, as this accounts for the longer ulnae that will cause these lifters to have a longer transition phase from the second pull to overhead, which results in more energy and effort expended. Shorter-stature and shorter-armed lifters will benefit from the elbow-to-elbow approach.

92. B: While body fat percentages can vary among individuals, a body fat percentage of 23% for a female athlete falls into the average range. 12% would be extremely low for a female and would potentially be too low for the body's essential fat stores, and 35% would be a higher amount of body fat than average.

93. B: Ketosis can be detrimental for an athlete, as the body needs significantly higher levels of energy substrate to perform higher-intensity or long-duration activities, and the supply of energy from ketosis will not provide adequate energy substrate for optimal performance levels. Transitioning into this state due to a low-carbohydrate diet can affect performance by reducing physical endurance, mental focus, cognitive function, and the ability to produce maximal muscular contractions for absolute strength purposes or high-velocity muscle activities such as sprinting or jumping.

94. A: Females of childbearing age are one of the groups most susceptible to iron deficiency. They have a greater need for iron, partly due to blood lost during the menstrual cycle.

95. B: Carbohydrate loading is a performance technique that increases stored muscle glycogen by consuming higher amounts of carbohydrates in the days leading up to an event. Eating more carbohydrates can be done at each meal and can include a balance of low-GI and high-GI carbohydrates, not just low-GI ones.

96. A: In the supine knee flex stretch, the athlete lays on their back and pulls one knee toward the chest by placing both hands behind the thigh. This stretches the hip extensors, which are the gluteals and hamstrings.

97. C: In an anxiety disorder, persistent feelings of worry or dread are so pervasive that they interfere with regular functioning, hindering the ability to focus or perform well.

98. B: Doing the side quadriceps stretch effectively requires holding a position that lengthens the quadriceps while avoiding any other extra movement or compensation (such as extending the lumbar spine or the thoracic spine).

99. A: Reduced resting heart rate is a primary chronic aerobic training adaptation. This occurs because of the stretching of the left ventricle over time, which increases the volume of blood ejected per contraction of the heart but causes a reduction in the frequency of contraction. This can result in bradycardia, which is a resting heart rate of 40–60 beats per minute.

100. C: Bronchioles are found in both the conduction and respiration zones. The respiratory bronchioles are responsible for approximately 10% of gas exchange during respiration. The division of the terminal bronchioles represents the end of the conduction zone in human respiration and can be identified with the occurrence of alveoli, which represents the beginning of the respiration zone.

101. A: Compound movements affecting large muscle groups coupled with higher loading intensities will result in the highest growth hormone release.

102. C: A triceps extension is an example of a first-class lever. The elbow is the axis (fulcrum) of the lever, the load (weight) is in the hand, and the triceps attach on the outer surface of the elbow, on the other side of the axis. Dumbbell lateral raises and biceps curls are both examples of third-class levers.

103. B: Warm-up movements for testing should mimic the needs of the test at lower intensity and include movements to prepare muscles for the ranges of motion in testing. The pro-agility test involves starting in a 3-point stance, and the forward lunge with elbow to instep is a dynamic stretch with similarities to this position. Walking knee lifts provide a dynamic stretch for the lower body as preparation for sprinting in the pro-agility test. Lastly, since the pro-agility test requires changing direction, low-intensity side shuffles allow practice of directional changes before implementing them at top speed.

104. C: Myosin ATPase, like other enzymes, is involved in a specific chemical reaction. Myosin ATPase is responsible for catalyzing the actomyosin cross-bridging response in muscular contraction.

105. C: An electrocardiogram (ECG) is used to assess the electrical signals generated during polarization and depolarization of cardiac tissue, which provides insight into the overall function and health of an athlete's heart. This test assesses the rate and frequency of the heartbeats while also determining the size and position of the heart's chambers. Assessing cardiovascular health in athletes is of extreme importance when considering issues like left ventricular hypertrophy, congenital heart defects, or other cardiac rhythm distortions that may cause health complications or even sudden death.

106. B: Whole practice refers to doing a specific skill or movement in its entirety rather than breaking it down into subcomponents, which is termed part practice. While there are many skills where whole practice and part practice can both be used, skills with highly related components are better learned through whole practice. A vertical jump would not be logical to separate into smaller components, as it would make the jump less effective. Therefore, the athlete is best off just practicing jumping.

107. A: In vicarious experience, a person observes others to model how actions should be done, facilitating understanding and familiarity before trying the actions themselves. This enhances self-efficacy (a situationally specific confidence in one's own abilities) because watching others do the drills successfully helps build confidence in the viewer's own ability to accomplish them.

108. A: An athlete using 50–60% of his 1-RM will be able to accelerate the barbell at the desired speed of approximately 0.08 m/s to facilitate an increase in speed. This percentage of the 1-RM is heavy enough to require a high force output from the athlete without risking muscular failure and allows for sufficient training volumes to develop the neurological consistency needed to increase the rate of signaling to the muscles to facilitate the increase in bar speed and, over time, speed in competition.

109. B: An athlete needing to improve a muscular weakness or increase the size of a muscle group would benefit significantly in a brief period from using a compound set approach for the affected muscle. Performing multiple movements in sequence to target the muscle group will not require the body to respond to significantly greater stresses to the body. This method is primarily oriented to force the muscle to work for longer periods of time under limited recovery conditions between movements to increase nutrient delivery to the training muscle. This increase in blood flow to the muscle will promote growth via increased local protein synthesis and, when coupled with heavier training methods in the early part of the training session, will allow the athlete to meet the training goal within the 4–6-week training block.

110. B: Core movements are compound movements that affect multiple joints and affect large muscle areas across the body. Structural movements are also multi-joint exercises and affect large muscle areas but are specifically movements that load the spine directly (e.g., a back squat) or indirectly (e.g., a power clean).

111. B: Higher-intensity activities increase the surface area of the neuromuscular junction and the length of nerve terminal branching and increase and disperse more widely the available synapse locations. These alterations in morphology indicate that with anaerobic training, neural transmission can be improved.

112. C: Decision-making skills, such as using a coach command (for example, directing the athlete to run left or right) use qualities of perceptual-cognitive ability, which include decision-making, accuracy, and reaction time. Using these types of qualities is essential for training agility; otherwise, the drill is simply a change of direction skill.

113. B: Having a gradual and highly structured approach to training load increases throughout a training program will ensure consistent results and allow athletes to achieve their primary resistance training goals in each sport season. Using an approach such as the two-for-two rule provides structure for gradual training load increases by requiring the athlete to perform two additional repetitions at an assigned training load above the prescribed repetitions during the final set and being able to achieve this result in two consecutive training sessions. Once this has been achieved, the training load will increase.

114. A: The barbell row does not occur in a prone position, the bar does not move overhead, and the spine is not directly loaded by the barbell. The athlete can safely execute the lift on the platform and abandon the lift, if necessary, without fear of injury or being unable to complete the lift. It is important to note that the trainer must always be alert, even if they are not technically spotting.

115. B: Lower body plyometric intensity levels are established by assessing the metabolic and neural demands placed on the athlete's body. Jumps that require lower force levels to generate the movement are of lowest impact, while jumps that require higher force levels are of higher impact.

116. B: The sarcoplasmic reticulum is a system of tubules surrounding each myofibril and is responsible for pumping calcium ions (Ca^{+}) into the muscle when an action potential releases onto the sarcomere. The sarcoplasmic reticulum is responsible for pumping calcium ions into the muscle to generate a contraction but is also the site of calcium ion storage. Without these essential functions, muscular contraction would not occur.

117. B: Muscle dysmorphia is a psychological condition also termed *reverse anorexia nervosa* that occurs when someone muscular has an altered self-image of being too small. Individuals with muscle dysmorphia continually seek to increase their muscle mass and may use anabolic steroids to help accomplish this.

118. B: Tests that are strenuous or high-intensity, such as 1-RM testing, place high demands on the cardiovascular system and should be avoided for any individual with cardiac issues, such as hypertension.

119. A: Complex training is combining a reactive stretch-shortening cycle exercise, such as a depth jump for height, and a traditional strength exercise in a similar movement pattern, such as the squat. Utilizing a complex training method, the athlete will benefit from the manipulation of the stretch-shortening cycle by increasing power via elastic energy recovery, increased movement efficiency, and rate of neural signaling through feedback and impulse strength.

120. B: Negligence refers to the failure of an individual to respond to a situation in an expected, logical manner and as a person with similar training and background would respond under similar circumstances. The importance of clearly outlining the emergency care plan is to establish the responsibilities and expectations of the staff members in the training facility. This can significantly mitigate problems that could arise regarding negligence or violation of the standard of care expectations for people who should have the essential knowledge and understanding of how to handle challenging emergency situations.

121. A: Contracting the agonist (in this case, the quadriceps, which is the agonist of the hamstrings) during the passive phase of a PNF stretch helps enhance the effectiveness of stretching through promoting reciprocal inhibition, which stimulates the Golgi tendon organ (GTO) in the hamstrings and causes further relaxation of the muscle.

122. A: The athlete has scored highly in two low-speed strength movements, indicating that they likely have the high level of requisite strength to also score highly on the power clean, especially since the two other movements require leg strength and pulling strength, which are also directly relevant to the power clean; however, since the power clean is a more technical movement, the lower percentile score suggests that the athlete may not yet be proficient in proper technique.

123. A: Athletes in strength and power sports benefit from consuming protein after resistance training, since this increases protein synthesis in the muscles, promoting recovery and potentially additional muscle hypertrophy.

124. C: In the stretch-shortening cycle, the muscles store energy as they are stretched and then rapidly release the energy through powerfully contracting. At maximal velocity, this is happening repeatedly with every stride and at a higher frequency than at acceleration or deceleration.

125. C: A comparative strength analysis is not essential when initiating a training program, as a comparison of strength levels between two athletes does not provide important information when establishing the core needs of an athlete in order to develop a training program. When performing an assessment on an individual athlete, the key elements to include are the needs analysis, movement and injury analysis, and evaluating training status and background, along with physiological assessments (strength, endurance, etc.).

126. A: The muscle spindle is the primary proprioceptive feedback structure in the muscle and the most important component in the stretch reflex response. The muscle spindle senses when a rapid stretch is applied to a muscle and reflexively contracts, which serves to potentiate the force-generating capacity of the muscle as well.

127. C: An athlete training in the 80% loading intensity range should generally be able to perform eight repetitions. Using a percentage of the 1-repetition maximum chart will provide significant guidance for assigning training load intensities when working in specific repetition ranges. For example, an athlete can be assigned to use a training load intensity prescription of 75–83% when assigned 7–10 repetitions per set, according to the 1-repetition maximum chart.

128. C: Counterconditioning uses a combination of somatic and cognitive techniques to reduce an athlete's performance-related anxiety. This is achieved through systematic desensitization that requires an athlete to engage in visualization of a stressful competitive situation. To counter the stress response, the athlete engages in progressive muscle relaxation to induce a relaxed mental and physical state.

129. A: For an athlete who has just completed an agility-focused training block, strength will necessarily need to be trained in the next block. This will also allow the progress made during the agility training block to manifest and continue to improve via enhanced neural connections, but increases in strength from the current training block will also play a role. Sequenced training is intended to develop multiple characteristics separately while also relying on the relationships between characteristics to develop the athlete's capacities.

130. C: The assistant strength and conditioning coach will possess many of the same responsibilities as the strength and conditioning director but may not directly oversee the training and development of as many athletic teams. The assistant strength and conditioning coach should achieve and maintain the necessary certification credentials, as the assistant and the strength and conditioning director are subject to the same facility or university professional standards and guidelines.

131. C: The Valsalva maneuver is appropriate to use with athletes who have been properly trained on movement skill and execution and those who have substantial training experience. Structural exercises that load the spine will require the use of the Valsalva maneuver in some cases to stabilize the spine properly when under heavy training loads. It is important to note that the Valsalva maneuver can lead to a loss of consciousness and requires extreme caution.

132. B: The main feature of variable practice is having changing practice conditions instead of isolating single skills. In this example, the athlete must repeatedly change the conditions of their basketball shot in the drill rather than focus on one type of shot. Repetitive-part training would have an athlete practice part of a skill in isolation, which is not occurring here. Simplification would change the task difficulty to make it easier than the normal task in the sport, like moving more slowly or having no defenders.

133. C: Using a body part split in an athletic training program is usually not the most effective method for developing an athlete. Body part split training requires limiting training frequency and the movements used. Power and structural movements require large muscle groups to work together and are difficult to segment according to predominant muscle activity. An athlete who is returning from an injury or is currently rehabilitating an injury can benefit from training the body parts, as this will allow the athlete to train around an injured area and still train non-affected muscles and joints. This approach will result in better results than rehabilitation or avoiding training.

134. A: While there is no single explanation for the significant association between eating disorders and anxiety and depressive disorders, individuals may use disordered eating to cope with negative feelings. Furthermore, individuals with disordered eating behaviors may struggle with a sense of low self-worth.

135. B: The endomysium encapsulates each muscle fiber. The perimysium is a layer of connective tissue that groups individual muscle fibers into fascicles. The epimysium is a sheath of dense connective tissue that covers the entire muscle, including the perimysium and endomysium, and is continuous with the fascia.

136. A: The strength and conditioning director is responsible for the selection of the equipment for purchase. This is due to the strength and conditioning director's expertise and understanding of the athletic needs of the program participants. Of the options listed, he is the only one who will have this unique qualification and authority. This does not mean, however, that he has the final word on whether the equipment is purchased; budgetary constraints may limit the strength and conditioning director's options, but this is an area where communication between staff members is essential.

137. A: Actin is a thin filament that is arranged in a double helix shape. It serves as the binding site for myosin, which, through ATP hydrolysis, generates a power stroke that causes the actin filament to slide past the myosin filament. The movement of actin and myosin is the basis of the sliding filament theory of muscular contraction.

138. B: Type I fibers are slow oxidative (i.e., slow-twitch) fibers that are primarily engaged in long-duration activities, as these fibers produce low levels of force and are fatigue resistant. Type IIa fibers are considered fast oxidative and glycolytic, are fast-twitch, produce medium amounts of force, and are highly fatigue resistant. Type IIb are considered fast glycolytic, are fast-twitch, produce large amounts of force, and are rapidly fatigued.

139. A: A preparatory routine is a process routine whereby an athlete undertakes specific steps to focus on a specific task. This routine allows an athlete to focus on an immediate task that effectively limits their exposure to elements that can negatively affect performance. This routine establishes a consistent approach to stressful situations and allows the athlete to perform consistently.

140. B: During spinal flexion, the rectus abdominis acts as the agonist and the erector spinae acts as the antagonist by stretching to accommodate the forward torso flexion. A muscle that is acting as an antagonist during a movement is performing a protective action, as the antagonist muscle groups are working to decelerate a force acting on the body while also stabilizing the working joints.

141. C: The proper starting position for the snatch requires the athlete to have their feet either hip or shoulder-width apart, the hips down below the shoulders, a grip that is wider than the snatch rings, elbows fully extended, and feet flat on the floor. The body is positioned with the back flat or slightly arched, chest held up and out, head in line with the vertebral column, heels on the floor, shoulders over or slightly in front of the bar, and eyes focused straight ahead or slightly upward.

142. C: Interval training, which includes both high-intensity interval training (HIIT) and Fartlek ("speed play") training, involves alternating work and rest periods and is useful for improving VO_2 max, lactate threshold, and anaerobic metabolism. While HIIT makes use of short bursts of intense activity (at or above 90% of VO_2 max for 30–90 seconds) followed by short periods of complete rest, Fartlek training uses lower-intensity (70–90% of VO_2 max) activity alternating with lower-intensity recovery periods, such as a run and a walk. Fartlek training is unstructured, allowing the athlete to adjust the intensity and duration of each interval based on their own goals and how they feel during training. The athlete can avoid overtraining by slowing down as needed rather than sticking to a program that may be too intense. Steady state training, which consists of consistent, low- or moderate-intensity activity (50–70% of VO_2 max), is best for beginners who are not yet ready for higher-intensity activity.

143. C: The oxidative system is the primary energy production system at rest and during low-intensity exercise. This system can utilize all three macronutrients as substrates but is predominantly oriented to use fats while at rest (~70%) and carbohydrates during low to moderate exercise intensities.

144. C: Athletes who train with maximal or near-maximal lifting intensities will require longer recovery times between training sessions. This is necessary because of the neural and muscular fatigue that occurs when lifting at heavy training intensities.

145. B: An athlete who is training for repetitive explosive bouts in competition will need to train at a sufficient threshold to develop the power capacity required but will also need to do so in a moderate fashion to be able to perform the activity at a high level over time. Training in the 75–85% loading intensity range meets the first requirement of using a training load that will require the athlete to move with great force and velocity, and the 3–5 repetitions per set is a sufficient amount of work per set to develop the capacity to produce large force and velocity consistently over a period.

146. B: The best test to assess an athlete's speed is the 150-meter sprint. When assessing an athlete's maximal speed, the testing procedure requires a straight line on a flat surface, with the final distance not surpassing the 200-meter mark. The reasoning behind limiting the distance of the testing procedure is because going beyond 200 meters becomes a test of anaerobic capacity and not straight-line maximal velocity. The additional distance violates the purpose and focus of the testing procedure.

147. C: After evaluating an athlete's balance, strength, and speed, the coach should evaluate the athlete's jumping technique, as this is necessary to develop a plyometric program. If the coach is not aware of movement errors in the athlete's jump, then the training program will not be successful.

148. A: Strength and conditioning professionals should be equipped and prepared to respond to emergencies, such as calling 911 or administering CPR, AED, or first aid, as this initial care can be lifesaving and is within the scope of practice of the role. While a strength and conditioning professional should use informed consent for their participants, it is not their duty to create the forms because they are legal documents. Clearance should only be done by a medical professional, such as a physician or physical therapist.

149. B: Selective attention refers to a person's ability to engage with the correct source of input while ignoring other forms of input. For an athlete, this means focusing on the performance tasks required during a competitive event while ignoring fans, loud noises, cheerleaders, players from the opposing team, etc. An athlete who has a high capacity to focus on the important aspects of performance will perform at a higher level than an athlete who struggles to handle excessive sensory inputs.

150. B: Hemoglobin is a combination molecule of iron and protein and is carried via red blood cells throughout the circulatory system of the human body. Hemoglobin serves as a transport system delivering oxygen to the body's tissues and carrying carbon dioxide away from tissues and back to the lungs, while also being responsible for buffering hydrogen ion concentrations in the blood.

151. B: In the provided list, the strength/power phase is representative of one of the alterations that have been made to Matveyev's model of periodization. The three alterations to the Matveyev model (the hypertrophy/endurance phase, the base strength phase, and the strength/power phase) occur during the preparation phase. Each training phase builds into the next, and each is defined by specific training load intensities and training volumes, with intensity increasing and training volume decreasing as the athlete moves from hypertrophy/endurance to strength/power.

152. C: Type I muscle fibers have the greatest capacity for morphological and physiological adaptations to aerobic training due to their higher initial oxidative capacity and the effect that training has on the size and number of mitochondria in the muscle cells along with the volume of circulating myoglobin. Type I muscle fibers have a higher initial oxidative capacity than type II fibers, which is and their capacity is increased more significantly by aerobic training than other muscle fiber type. Type I fibers will also hypertrophy in response to aerobic training, though not to the same degree as the type II fiber types when undertaking anaerobic training programs, such as resistance training and sprint conditioning programs.

153. C: Muscular plasticity is the capacity of a muscle to be gradually stretched to achieve a new and greater length after a passive or static stretching action. This allows for the stiffness in the athlete's hamstring to be reduced to manageable levels to facilitate a high level of performance and reduce apprehensions of sustaining an injury. Elasticity is the ability to return to a specific resting length after a passive stretching action.

154. A: The principle of progressive overload refers to a gradual increase in the amount of external resistance an athlete must work against during training-related activities. Overload can be achieved by increasing the number of repetitions per set with a specific resistance, increasing the volume of work performed in a training session or set period (supersets, compound sets, etc.), increasing the total number of sets performed at a specific loading parameter, and reducing rest periods, which is another form of increasing work density.

155. B: Determining an athlete's training status is the key element for determining training frequency. An athlete who does not have a significant training background will require fewer training sessions per week to facilitate improvements, while a more experienced and conditioned athlete will require greater frequency to stimulate progress.

156. C: When the athlete first contacts the ground, the agonist muscles are preloaded, storing elastic energy, and stimulate the muscle spindle (eccentric). After the muscles are preloaded and the energy has been stored, there is a momentary pause in muscle action (amortization). The briefer the amortization phase, the greater the stored energy release will be. If the amortization phase is too long, the energy will be significantly less. The final phase (concentric) occurs when the stored energy is released at the same time as the contraction of the affected muscles, which increases the force of the movement or is dissipated as heat.

157. C: Ergogenic aids are pharmacological substances used to augment physiological processes to enhance athletic performance. These substances can be used to enhance muscular recovery and metabolism or to increase circulating anabolic hormones. While acetaminophen can reduce inflammation of joints and other tissues, this will not help recovery, and current research indicates that using non-steroidal anti-inflammatory drugs after a training session can hinder physiological recovery.

158. A: The sinoatrial (SA) node generates the electrical signals that contract the heart and is commonly referred to as the "pacemaker" for this reason. The SA node is located in the right atrium and establishes the normal heart rhythm, which is referred to as the sinus rhythm.

159. C: Potentiation is a neurophysiological response that increases the contractile capacity of muscles via alteration of the force-velocity curve due to stretch, which also increases neural drive to the working muscles. Potentiation functions to increase the muscles' capacity for force production by generating a reflexive response from the nervous system that can be used to decrease recruitment thresholds for fast-twitch muscle fibers that are necessary to perform strength exercises at or above maximal intensity levels. Using this combined training approach can result in immediate strength increases for a training session and significantly affect strength progression over the course of several weeks.

160. B: The basic strength phase is the first phase when sport-specific and practice activities occur. This training phase is part of the preparation phase and occurs after the hypertrophy and endurance phase and is highlighted by high-intensity training loads and moderate training volumes. The emphasis of this training phase is to improve muscular strength for the primary muscles involved in the sport-specific movements the athlete will need to perform at the highest level possible.

161. A: Golgi tendon organs are responsible for inhibiting tension overload in muscle and tendons when placed under stretch. The Golgi tendon organ emits electrical signals from its sensory neuron to an inhibitory neuron in the spinal cord, which inhibits the motor neuron in the same muscle. This signaling process is very rapid and leads to an immediate reduction in tension within the muscle, preventing excessive loading injuries and even reactive stress injuries.

162. C: Of these options, anabolic steroids have the highest potential for adverse effects. They can affect many physiological systems, such as the cardiovascular system and the endocrine system. In addition, anabolic steroids can cause permanent changes to the genitals and cause psychological symptoms such as psychotic episodes and aggressive behavior.

163. B: If equipment limitations are an issue when testing maximal anaerobic power, the vertical jump is the most cost-effective method. To test the vertical jump, you need a wall, a measuring tape or stick, and chalk. To perform the test, the athlete stands flat-footed next to the testing wall and reaches to mark, in chalk, the highest point possible with the dominant arm. Once this has been completed, the athlete sets their feet, jumps as high as possible, and sets another chalk mark. After the two marks have been set, the measurement can be taken to assess the height of the jump.

164. C: The American College of Sports Medicine standard for the push-up assessment is for the participant to perform as many repetitions as possible in a continuous fashion until failure. There is no time consideration for the testing procedure, and it is simply a test of local muscle endurance in the chest, shoulders, and triceps.

165. C: The recommended rest period for athletes training to enhance muscular endurance is ≤ 30 seconds between sets. This is intentional to perform large amounts of work in a brief period, which will enhance an athlete's ability to sustain effort over time. This is also a result of the percentage of 1-RM that is recommended, as lighter training loads ($< 70\%$) can be lifted for a higher total number of repetitions per set than heavier training loads.

166. A: Strength allows an athlete to overcome increased resistance generated on the body as acceleration occurs. The ability to overcome the force of gravity as movement velocity increases via greater force production through increased muscular contraction is essential for developing maximal linear speed but also significant for decelerating, changing directions, or leaping.

167. B: A full review of the strength and conditioning program should take place at the end of the competitive year, as the postseason period will consist of little training for the athletes other than general sport activity, and the next competitive season will not begin until the off-season training program begins again. The strength and conditioning coach should evaluate athlete progress over the course of each sport season, but a full qualitative review is not required until the end of the competitive season.

168. C: A very high range for VO_2 max is 63–69 mL/kg/min. Values in this range, or even higher, would be expected for an athlete in a long-distance, aerobic sport like cross-country, since the nature of the sport directly trains aerobic capacity.

169. C: Athletes have a higher protein need than the general population because of higher protein turnover rates, the need to maintain a positive nitrogen balance, and the need to facilitate recovery and restoration of working tissues. The general recommendation for daily protein intake for the average person is 0.8 g/kg of body weight, and athletes are advised to consume 1.4–1.8 g/kg of body weight.

170. C: Testosterone affects muscular physiology via increased protein synthesis and increased growth hormone production in the pituitary glands. Testosterone can also affect central nervous system adaptations to resistance training by increasing neuronal receptor activity, increasing neurotransmitter activity and availability, and altering structural proteins that facilitate muscular contraction.

171. B: When training individuals with limited training experience, the most important component for testing is to ensure maximal safety and to perform the test in such a way that the result is useful for multiple loading intensities. This requires the strength and conditioning professional to use a repetition maximum that is useful for moderate loading intensities while also being light enough to ensure technique and joint health are not compromised. Using a 6–8 repetition maximum is the most effective and safest option for an athlete with limited training experience.

172. A: A neutral spine should be maintained during a squat, which includes avoiding rounding or arching at the low back. Cueing the athlete to lift the chest helps avoid torso flexion, where the athlete leans forward instead of maintaining a neutral spine.

173. C: Myofibrils are the internal structure of the muscle fiber (myocyte) and contain the long, thin chains of protein responsible for contraction of the muscle fiber. Myofibrils are made up of long strands of the proteins actin, myosin, and titin. These proteins are arranged along the myofibril into thick and thin filaments, which are arranged into compartments known as sarcomeres. Muscle contraction takes place all along the myofibril as the actin filaments (thin filaments) slide along the length of the myosin (thick filaments), generating muscular contractions.

174. B: Performing a needs analysis is a two-step process that requires the strength and conditioning coach to evaluate the movements and physiological requirements for a specific sport and the needs of the individual athlete. This process ensures accuracy in addressing the essential needs of competition while also considering the specific needs of an individual athlete based on their injury history, training status, and physiological status.

175. B: The sarcolemma is essential in conducting and receiving stimuli from the connecting nerve fibers. The ability of the sarcolemma to transduce electrical signals allows the t-tubules that run from side to side throughout the sarcolemma to release Ca^{2+} ions into the sarcoplasm.

176. A: Training during the inflammatory phase of injury recovery is not a forbidden activity, but the training should be limited to the healthy joints and muscles. This may require using a body part split to avoid excessive loading in the injured area, such as squatting with a leg or hip injury. The key is to work to maintain strength and endurance at sufficient levels such that once the athlete is cleared to return to training or competitive activities, the athlete will not be as far away from top condition as if they were not to engage in any training at all.

177. C: Using variability to assess a large statistical sample is the best approach to evaluating the effectiveness of the program for the total group sample. Standard deviation will separate the data if the data is normal, which is most probable, according to the best and least responsive to the training program. This will provide clear insight into the global effectiveness of the program but not on an individual basis. A program may have some very poor performers, such as a college freshman with little training experience, who make substantial progress but are still considered below average according to a variability analysis.

178. B: Using a non-linear periodization model allows the strength and conditioning coach to vary training load intensities and training volumes according to the competition schedule, as there may be significant gaps between events that allow the athlete to increase intensity and training volume for a two- to three-week period, in a sort of peaking strategy, to make progress over previous competitions. This could also be used in a sport with weekly competitions, such as a collegiate football or gymnastics program, as this would allow the strength and conditioning coach to evaluate the needs of the athlete based on the difficulty of the upcoming meet or game and prescribe training volumes and training load intensities accordingly. This approach also allows for significant variation during each training week, as training load intensity and volume can be altered day to day if desired.

179. C: Erythropoietin is a protein hormone that stimulates the production of red blood cells. The suggested mechanism for enhancing aerobic endurance performance is increasing hemoglobin levels, the result of increased hematocrit and decreased plasma volume. The decrease in plasma volume is thought to be caused by downregulation of the renin-angiotensin-aldosterone axis.

180. A: The semilunar valves, also known as the aortic and pulmonary valves, are responsible for preventing backflow into the ventricles during ventricular relaxation (diastole). This function is passive, as these valves open and close based on the directional pressures produced by the heart. Backward pressure causes the valves to close, while forward pressure opens the valves to allow movement of blood out of the ventricles.

181. C: Any non-fatiguing tests, such as a vertical jump, should go first in a test battery. Agility tests require high levels of skill and neuromuscular control and should precede tests for maximal power and strength, such as 1-RM tests. Otherwise, fatigue from the 1-RM might impair agility performance.

182. A: When training for muscular hypertrophy, the outlined criteria call for as few repetitions as 6 per set and as many as 12. The suggested number of sets falls between 3 and 6 total sets. An athlete who performs 5 sets of 10 repetitions will perform 50 total repetitions of a given movement, which will result in the highest training volume of the options listed and will cause the greatest change in muscular hypertrophy over time.

183. B: The parasympathetic nervous system is responsible for relaxation or periods of decreased activity levels that govern various passive activities such as digestion. A high activity level in this division of the autonomic nervous system would be detrimental to competition because this system decreases mental acuity, focus, heart rate, and other physiological processes that need to be at heightened activity levels to respond to the competitive environment.

184. C: The correct hierarchy for developing speed and agility is making sure to properly orient the methodology, which means establishing the primary, secondary, and tertiary methods for inclusion in the program. This would place primary methods first, which consist of sprint and agility training to acquire the correct technical skill and develop the basic patterns first in the training program. Secondary methods would include using specialized techniques to develop acceleration, maximal velocity, or other special skills and utilizing sprint assistance or sprint resistance techniques to achieve this end. The tertiary methods for developing an athlete's sprint and agility capacities would include mobility, strength, and endurance training.

185. A: The proper order in this example should begin with the pro-agility test, as this test relies on coordinated movement and therefore should occur before the athlete becomes fatigued due to the other testing procedures. The 1-RM squat test should occur next, as this is a maximum strength and power test and, likewise, must not occur after a test that causes excessive fatigue. The 110-meter sprint test should be next in the battery because this test requires the athlete to achieve maximal velocity; this test should not be placed after a test of local endurance, as fatigue accumulation would affect the testing procedure. The final test in the battery should be the local endurance test, as this test will accrue the highest localized muscular fatigue and would affect the other testing procedures if conducted earlier in the sequence. Proper testing order in a battery of tests is important, as activities that utilize differing energy systems or require significant levels of movement coordination create different types of fatigue that will limit performance on other tests when not sequenced correctly.

186. B: Extension of the hips, knees, and ankles, otherwise known as triple extension, occurs during the second pull of the Olympic lifts. This is the phase when the most rapid and explosive power is generated.

187. C: Improving the strength ratio at the affected joint where frequent injuries occur is a basic step in programming to correct a structural weakness. Addressing the issue after proper rehabilitative steps have been completed would consist of addressing the underlying deficiency through properly programming the resistance training for the athlete. In this example, the athlete would be required to focus on developing posterior strength and resiliency. This could be achieved through movement patterns that directly engage this area (e.g., deadlift, glute-ham raise, reverse hyperextension, step-ups, hip thrusts). A wide range of repetitions could be chosen, including strength emphasis work (e.g., 4–12 repetitions per set). This phase would also see a maintenance level of quad-dominant training prescribed, and for a period of four to six weeks could be eliminated to allow all training energies to be directed to correcting the imbalance.

188. A: A negligence claim could be brought against the strength and conditioning professional because they have failed to act with providing the expected standard of care of their role through obtaining a medical history for each participant to keep them safe and be aware of any contraindications for exercise. While the professional has neglected to do something important, they have not done something outside of their scope of practice (i.e., providing diagnosis, medical treatment, therapy, counseling, etc.). Assumption of risk refers to the participants being informed of the risks and choosing to participate, not action done by the professional.

189. A: The hold-relax with agonist contraction is the most effective form of PNF, as the added concentric contraction of the agonist promotes both reciprocal inhibition and autogenic inhibition.

190. C: Free weight pressing or pushing exercises, such as the dumbbell bench press or dumbbell shoulder press, should be spotted near the wrists. This places the spotter's hands closest to the dumbbells.

191. B: The RAMP protocol stands for Raise, Activate, Mobilize, Potentiate. The first step is getting the body temperature up via key movements (Raise), and the second step is improving overall movement capacity (Activate). The next step in a RAMP warm-up would be M for Mobilize. The purpose is to bring more mobility into key body segments, such as with dynamic stretches.

192. A: A physiological adaptation that allows for greater ATP production is the increased number of mitochondria in the muscle tissue. This alteration occurs because of the increased energy demands placed on the muscles due to the continuous aerobic endurance exercise or training. This change increases the availability of ATP in closest proximity to the working muscle tissues, which is a result of increased oxidation in the tissues.

193. B: Amphetamines are a type of stimulant. Stimulants speed up body processes through the central nervous system. Signs and symptoms include increased heart rate, increased sweating, and erratic or restless behavior.

194. C: The YMCA bench press test assesses upper body muscular endurance with a prescribed weight (80 lb [36 kg] for males and 35 lb [16 kg] for females) lifted at a specific tempo, 60 beats per minute. The pace is kept by a metronome. The bar is lifted on one beat and lowered on the next beat. This continues until the athlete cannot maintain this pace.

195. A: During anaerobic glycolysis, the energy system that is active when oxygen is not readily available, the pyruvate molecule will undergo fermentation, via lactate dehydrogenase and coenzyme NADH, to lactate to produce sufficient ATP. If oxygen is present, aerobic glycolysis will take place through oxidative phosphorylation, which requires pyruvate to enter the mitochondrion of a cell and then, when oxygen is present, is oxidized and enters the Krebs cycle.

196. C: A typical structure for HIIT use in aerobic conditioning is to intersperse higher-intensity work periods of 30–90 seconds with an equal amount of rest, though the rest can be longer (up to a ratio of 1:5) to keep each interval at top effort. Ratios of 1:12 to 1:20 would be most appropriate for anaerobic conditioning, not aerobic, such as training the phosphagen system through short bursts of near-maximal speed with substantial recovery time.

197. A: Guided discovery provides general instructions on a task without specific rules. This cue allows the athlete to discover for themself what body position might be necessary to accomplish the task as the coach has directed. Cueing feet pressing evenly is an example of intrinsic feedback, where the athlete uses their own sensory information to help with accomplishing the task. Deadlifting at a slower pace using a light weight like an empty bar would be an example of simplification, not guided discovery.

198. A: Cartilaginous joints are tough, fibrous joints between two bones. They allow movement that is primarily intended to allow the body flexibility and elasticity, such as during growth or respiration. Primary cartilaginous joints, or synchondroses, include growth plates (which are absent in adults) and the first sternocostal joint. Secondary cartilaginous joints, or symphyses, are permanent joints along the skeletal midline. These include the pubic symphysis and intervertebral discs. Synovial joints, or diarthroses, are freely moving capsulated joints between adjacent bones. There are six types of synovial joints, classified based on their physical shape and whether they are uniaxial (which move in one plane) or multiaxial (which move in multiple planes). These types are plane joints, hinge joints, pivot joints, condyloid joints, saddle joints, and ball-and-socket joints.

199. A: In pure-part training, parts of a skill are performed separately before combining them. In this case, the gymnast practicing each of the three components in their routine segment before putting them all together fluidly is an example of pure-part training. This is not random practice, as the skills are not done in a random order, and it is not explicit instructions, as the scenario does not provide any prescriptive information on how the coach gives details on the movement or sequence.

200. B: The most effective approach for reporting the times to the athletes is to take the average of the 12 timers because the sample size is small and removing any score will affect the accuracy of the reporting, as the differences between the lowest and highest score should be minimal. Scores should not be removed unless they are off by more than one second when compared to the other scores, which could indicate user error during measurement.

201. C: The athlete's score is the best of three trials to the nearest 0.5 inches or 1 cm for standing long jump and vertical jump. In addition, a countermovement is part of proper technique, and ground contact time is not measured for these tests.

202. C: Immediately after the backward movement phase where hip flexion is used to swing the kettlebell between the legs, a powerful drive from hip extension and knee extension propels the kettlebell forward in the upward movement phase.

203. C: To accurately collect testing data over a period, testing conditions must be similar to the original testing period. Adverse testing conditions (e.g., extreme temperature or rainy weather) will affect the athlete being tested, as will testing on different ground surfaces. Another element for testing is to make sure that the athlete is properly hydrated and properly fed (i.e., not fasted or recently fed). Testing conditions should closely resemble each other as much as possible. While it is important to test regularly in order to track progress, this does not need to be on a strict schedule, nor does it need to be very frequent.

204. B: Electrolytes include sodium, potassium, and chloride. As these are lost during sweating, athletes who exercise for long periods should consume electrolytes (such as through a sports drink) to replenish them. Maintaining electrolytes during long-duration exercise also helps avoid hyponatremia, which is a dangerous condition when blood sodium falls too low.

205. C: Butter, other animal fats, and tropical oils like coconut oil and palm oil are high in saturated fats. Corn oil and soybean oil are high in polyunsaturated fats.

206. A: Diuretics are a class of drugs taken orally to change the balance of water in the body. While diuretics may be used for legitimate medical conditions like hypertension, their typical performance use is for losing weight; however, loss of weight through excreting excess body water poses a risk of dehydration.

207. A: The muscle spindle is responsive to rapid changes in muscle length. When activated, the muscle spindle will cause a reflexive muscle action called the stretch reflex in the affected muscle or muscle group. This actually inhibits the muscle from relaxing and lengthening and would be counterproductive for stretching.

208. B: A starting position with shoulders over the bar or slightly in front of the bar for the Olympic lifts helps ensure that the first pull will be effective, with adequate power generation for the second pull.

209. C: Intrinsic feedback comes from an internal source, namely the athlete's own senses, rather than an outside source, such as an app or a coach's direction. In this scenario, the athlete uses their sense of sight to observe their knee alignment in the mirror.

210. C: Stride frequency is the primary determinant of an athlete's maximal velocity. As speed reaches maximal velocity, stride length tends to stabilize, meaning that any increases in velocity are largely the result of increased stride frequency.

211. A: The sticking point is the transition point between the eccentric and concentric movements. This point can occur exactly at this moment of transition or slightly above or below this transition depending on the movement pattern or an athlete's specific muscular weaknesses. It is important to note that the Valsalva maneuver can lead to a loss of consciousness and requires extreme caution.

212. B: A contusion is a trauma that occurs in the muscles and the tendons of the affected muscle. A contusion occurs because of direct trauma, usually a heavy impact or sudden, excessive stretching of the muscle, and results in the accumulation of blood and fluid in the tissues surrounding the injured area. This injury occurs as a result of an external force and is not a result of overuse or overtraining.

213. A: In part practice, a skill or movement is broken down into parts that are then practiced individually, such as the arm stroke practiced separately from the leg stroke during swimming. Sprinting and mobility techniques are not examples of part practice, as they do not break movements down into smaller components for the purposes of learning or improving technique.

214. C: For most efficient movement and maximal force generation in the snatch, the hips and shoulders should rise at the same time, keeping the angle of the torso constant relative to the floor.

215. B: The RAMP protocol is a common and effective protocol used for warm-ups that progresses through Raising body temperature, Activating and Mobilizing the body through sport-specific movement patterns and full ranges of motion (such as dynamic stretches), and using Potentiation to increase the intensity of sports-specific activities.

216. B: Blood doping is a banned method of performance enhancement that involves increasing the amount of red blood cells in the body, either through using a hormone (erythropoietin) or receiving blood transfusions. Since red blood cells carry oxygen, increasing them through these artificial methods will increase the body's oxygen utilization.

217. B: Weight trees should be limited to a distance of 36 inches from the lifting area. This will allow space between the equipment area and the plate storage area so that the loading and unloading of plates will not be hindered by limited space and will also help to expedite the loading and unloading process by having the necessary space to move the necessary tonnage to and from the training area. This will ensure the safety of the athletes when loading and unloading plates during training.

218. C: The strength and conditioning coach will have most frequent contact with the sports physical therapist or the athletic trainer. Communication between members of the medical team is essential, and the strength and conditioning coach must stay in frequent contact with the sports physical therapist or athletic trainer. Players of any sport will have injuries, and communicating the athletes' needs is of the greatest importance. Proper communication between the physical therapist/athletic trainer and the strength and conditioning coach ensures that an athlete will not just to be able to play in the next game but also for the athlete to effectively heal and strengthen the affected joint or muscle over time.

219. C: Optimal sprinting technique is highly dependent on the correct application of force into the ground. Keeping the ground contact time (the amount of time that the feet are in contact with the ground) minimal promotes the development of explosive strength, which in turn increases sprint speed.

220. B: Regularly using substances, such as alcohol, to cope with emotions is a possible indicator of a substance use disorder. Daily use can lead to becoming physically and/or psychologically dependent on the substance.

Online Resources

Due to our efforts to try to keep this book to a manageable length, we've created a link that will give you access to all of your online resources:

mometrix.com/resources719/cscs-31572

It's Your Moment, Let's Celebrate It!

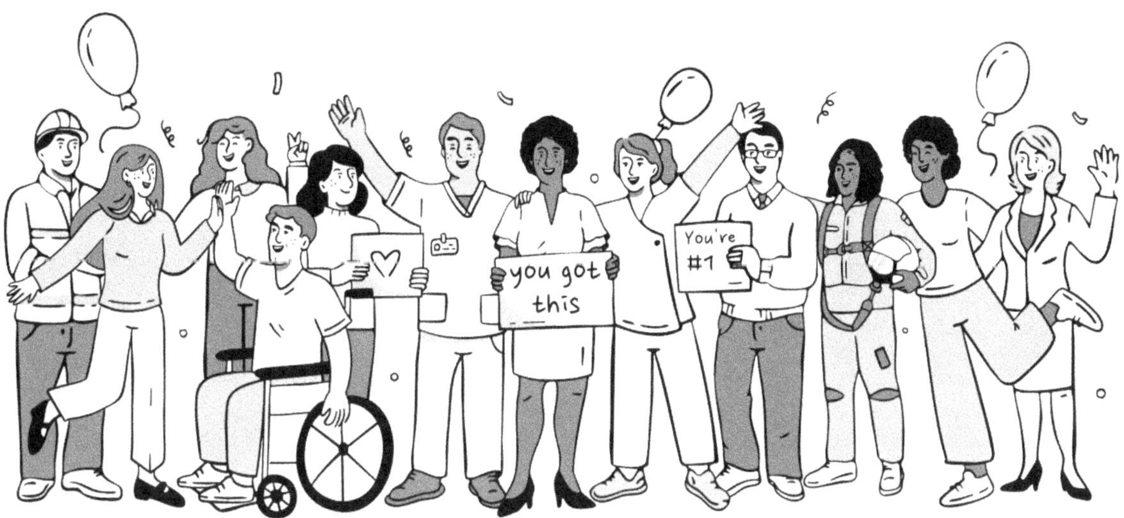

Share your story @mometrixtestpreparation

www.ingramcontent.com/pod-product-compliance
Lightning Source LLC
LaVergne TN
LVHW061241100826
845148LV00008B/1004
* 9 7 8 1 5 1 6 7 3 1 5 7 2 *